# IGNITE WELLNESS

# Open to Joy

A guide to integrate more health & happiness into your daily lifestyle.

**HEATHER NADINE LENZ**

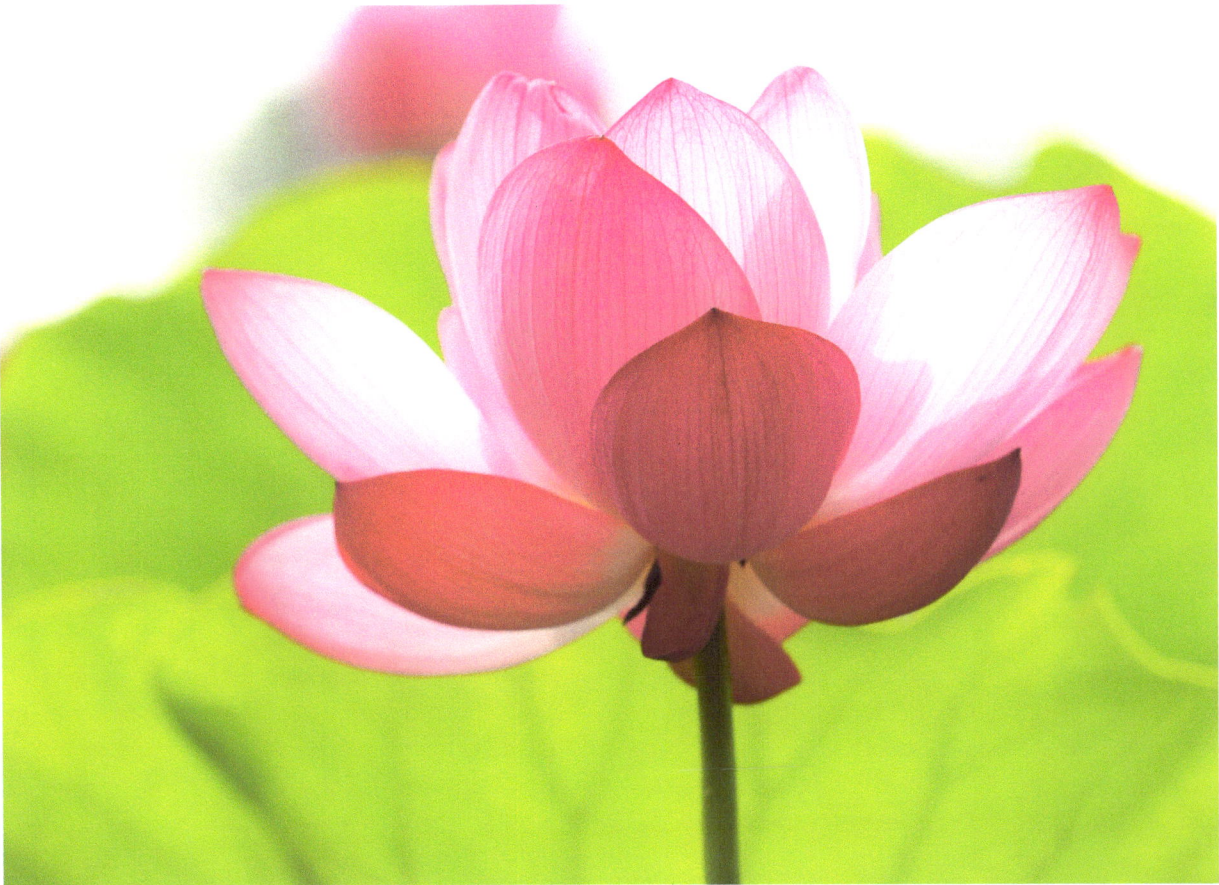

"When you make the present moment, instead of past and future, the focal point of your life, your ability to enjoy what your do - and with it the quality of your life - increases dramatically. Joy is the dynamic aspect of Being."

~ ECKHART TOLLE

**Ignite Wellness, Open to Joy**
Heather Nadine Lenz

Plum Tree Publishing

Published in the United States by Plum Tree Press

Conceived, created, and designed by Heather Nadine Lenz and Plum Tree Press.

Copyright © Heather Nadine Lenz

Managing Editor: Anna Brown
Text Editor: John Green
Designer: Heather Nadine Lenz

Library of Congress Cataloging-in-Publication is available

ISBN: 978-0-9980129-4-0

Typeset in Helvetica Neue and Helvetica Ultralight

**Notes**

Before following the advice or exercise in this book, we recommend that you ask your doctor whether it is suitable for you, especially if you suffer from any health disorders or special conditions. The publisher and author cannot accept any responsibility for any injuries or damage incurred as a result of the exercises in this book, or of using any of the therapeutic methods described or mentioned here.

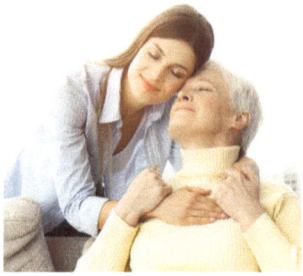

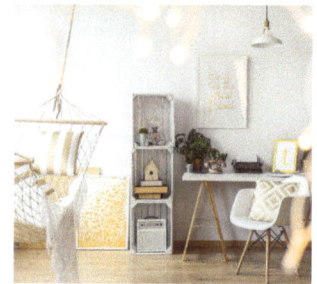

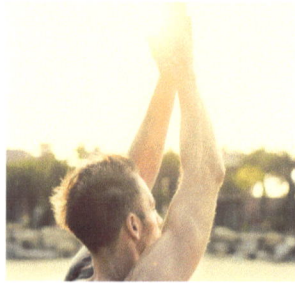

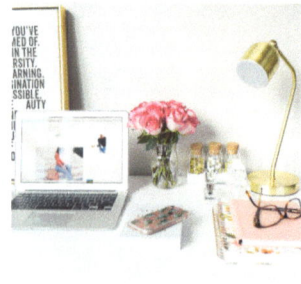

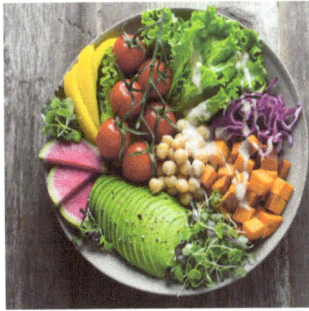
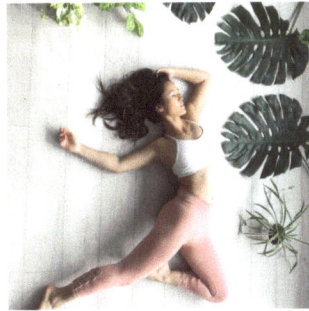
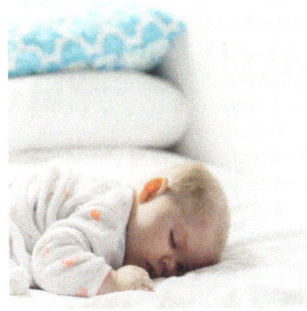
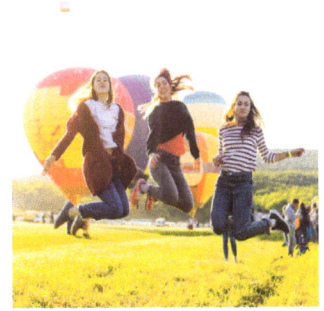

# Infusing wellness into your daily life.

A complete guide to integrate health & wellness into your daily lifestyle.

The intention of this book is to infuse more wellness into your everyday life and inspire you to open to joy. Inspiration is beautiful, but no one's life changes without taking action.

Therefore I give practical techniques and practices you can use right away to make a quantum leap in your physical, mental, and spiritual health. Seeking balance on all levels of being will activate your wellness, happiness and vitality.

Each section walks you through how to add more wellness to different parts of your day, from waking in the morning until drifting into slumber at night. Small changes in the way you live your daily life can cause a radical difference in your well-being.

The most significant change is focusing on channeling more love to flow in, through, and from you. Starting your day with the MORNING REVITALIZE program is the cornerstone for elevating how good you feel in your body, mind, and spirit. You will start your day feeling energized, balanced, supple, and inspired. Working with intention, focus, and creativity at work will become increasingly effortless as you implement the practices in the work section. Negative stress will melt away and you will be able to leverage positive stress to accomplish the results you desire.

In the Homemaking and Care giving sections you will discover how to amplify the wellness of your home and how to bring more wellness into your life as a caregiver.

Learning to eat and drink fresh, colorful food mindfully can change your health, well-being, and spark joy. A new approach to eating begins by blessing whatever food is in front of you with gratitude and asking that it nourish your body with vital health.

The after work relaxation section asks you to turn off all things digital and begin to treat life like a verb again. After you melt away any lingering stress and fatigue with breath work and yoga, then it's time to meditate, get out in nature, dance, move, learn, play, create, read or socialize.

Optimum wellness is impossible without sleep. The sleep section reveals how you can optimize your going-to-bed routine to get higher quality slumber.

Discovering your unique dosha compilation will equip you with the ability to act to bring yourself back into balance and radiant health in body and mind.

The final section of this book reveals how you can approach your weekends in a new way to uplift, rejuvenate, inspire, and make your next work week more successful. Taking time to become still, to reflect, and to plan out our time according to our values can enable us to make a quantum leap in life quality.

## HOW TO USE THIS BOOK

You can read through this like a regular book, but far better is to use it as an action guide. Always check with your doctor first, then introduce one section into your life each month. Remain positive if you miss a day. Just return to infusing wellness into your life in the next moment. Be a detective searching for what works and feels best for your unique body, mind, life situation, and soul. Allow yourself to redefine what you enjoy and what you are capable of achieving. Dream big and feel the emotions of having wellness in all areas of your life.

What does your ideal life feel like in your body? Then return again and again to right now, to what action you can take at this moment. Feel gratitude and pride in the areas of your life where you feel wellness and joy. Seek with equanimity to infuse more well-being and happiness into parts of your daily life that need your attention.

What I know for sure is that we are ALL challenged with some area of our wellness. I know I am! I am on this wellness journey with you. Seeking perfection is an impossible game. Instead, pursue bringing yourself back into balance over and over again.

Imagine yourself on a surfboard. When waves of stress, life situations, or negative emotions flow toward you, then you may start to waver, shake, or almost fall. Pause. Observe your thoughts and feelings. Inhale deeply through the nose to the count of three. Exhale as slowly as you can out the mouth to the count of eight. Feel into your body by bringing your awareness from the top of your head through to the tips of your toes.

Allow any emotions to be without acting on them, then take a healthy action from your joy or well-being list to bring yourself back into balance.

Wishing you radiant wellness and joy - Heather

*"Believe nothing, no matter where you read it, or who said it, no matter if I have said it, unless it agrees with your own reason and your own common sense." -Buddha*

# Opening to Joy

How much of the time is the authentic YOU showing up in the world? Do you have a different persona for your work, home life, friends, strangers, and the check-in person at the airport?

Stress, grief, past or current pain or trauma, illness, or anxiety can cause us to retreat inward.

Just like preparing a house to survive the impact of a hurricane, we can close the shutters, protect fragile points of entry, conserve resources, stock up on necessities, and retreat inside.

If you have found yourself hiding the real you from the world, don't worry. You're not alone. Unless you are age four or under, crafting an ever-shifting-persona is a natural protection mechanism. We learn as we grow-up that opening up and being authentic can lead to a slug of pain and a slap of heartache. Intuitively we find out what psychologists have tested to be true: people like those who mimic or mirror their body language. People also find it easier to like those who are similar or share the same interests and passions. So is it any wonder that all at once everyone is wearing the same color of teal or using the same slang? Is it a surprise that individuals in a group can converge in dress, tastes, interests, and values? The question is: do you want to open up and be more yourself at the risk of getting hurt and allowing people to release from your life? How much do you want to open to joy?

*"There are only two ways to live your life. One is as though nothing is a miracle. The other is as though everything is a miracle." – Albert Einstein*

## Step 1: Find Your Joy

Can you name five concrete experiences that bring you joy? Joy is delight fused with serenity and evokes a sense of connection to others, nature, or the divine. Joy is playful and generous.

The first step towards opening up and being authentically you is to uncover what brings you joy. List at least five experiences which bring joy into your life on a daily basis.

Next, you can explore and remember what caused a flash of unexpected joy in the past few months. Recall moments of bliss from your life and write them down too. List at least five surprises which bring joy into your life sporadically.

Be warned against ascribing to your cultural or familial imprinted definitions of delight. Whereas joy for everyone around you could be a rainbow sprinkled ice-cream cone, for you, it could be a cup of tea and dramatic rainclouds shifting across the sky.

**Looking for some joy-list inspiration? Here's my list:**

The first sip of espresso in the morning in my garden
Strolling barefoot on the dew-covered grass
A baby or child laughing
A bright dash of color. White and blank space
Smiling at someone I don't know on my walk
Hugs
Listening to my sleeping children
Settling into a smooth writing flow
Sliding into clean sheets with a captivating book
The last ten minutes of yoga when you melt into bliss
Stopping to admire the view on a hike up a mountain
Jumping into the waters of a clear, cold lake
Falling into the arms of a beloved after time apart
Dressing up to celebrate
Mastering a new skill for the first time
Laying on my back in the grass, watching the clouds
Going dancing. Being silly
Cutting and arranging fresh cut flowers
Giving the perfect gift or experience
Hugging a tree in the woods
Feeling sunlight warm on my skin

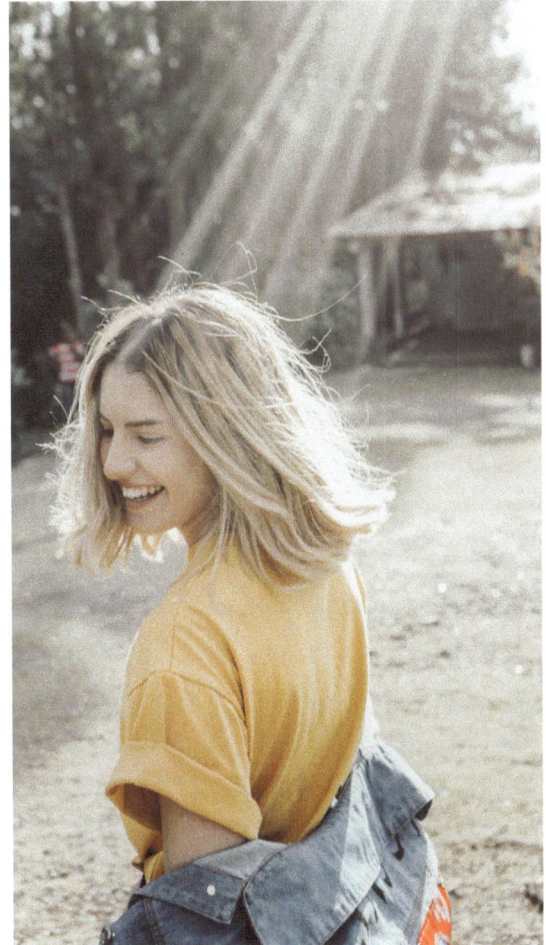

*"When you sparkle, you inspire others to do the same." - Doreen Virtue*

## Step 2: Schedule in More Joy Moments

It turns out, you can add more joy to your life at little cost. By scheduling more of what brings YOU joy into your life, you will be illuminating the authentic you; you'll begin to be more of you with everyone, everywhere you go.

The truth is that joy is contagious. The positive energy bounces off you and out into the world. People around you will feel your 'good vibrations' and respond with a smile. Unless they are grumpy sour-faces. Then they will resent you like hell until of course, they ask you why you are so damn happy. In which case, you can tell them. You can even show them your list, and ask them for their Joy Top Five.

## Step 3: Relate in a New Way

When you meet someone new, which YOU do you present? What is the first question you ask? The first question a lot of people ask is, 'so, what do you do?' or 'what do you study?' or 'where are you from?' It is natural for all of us to be comparing. The ego likes to rank where we stand. We can have the very best intentions, but when we ask about someone's job, it will be challenging to resist ascribing judgment based on their profession.

When you meet someone new, which YOU do you present? What is the first question you ask? The first question a lot of people ask is, 'so, what do you do?' or 'what do you study?' or 'where are you from?' It is natural for all of us to be comparing. The ego likes to rank where we stand. We can have the very best intentions, but when we ask about someone's job, it will be challenging to resist ascribing judgment based on their profession. The same is true for where they come from too.

Try it. If I say that I'm an award-winning artist living in New York city, what happens? If I shift to telling you I'm studying astrophysics in Russia, what is your reaction? What about if I answer I am a housekeeper in England?

Now try asking someone about their sources of joy in their daily life. What will happen? They will most likely answer honestly. People don't tend to lie about what brings them delight. You can sense a genuine answer by the way their eyes light up when they talk about their source of joy.

Then you will either find out that you:

1.  Share a common source of joy

2. Discover something new and authentic about the person that creates a deeper connection.

3. Could try the idea yourself. Who knows, maybe YOU should schedule in time to drink cold champagne in the bath too.

## Step 4: Be Brave - Control the Conversation

Perhaps it's time to shift the conversation. The pressure of kicking-ass at work and adding being a source of support and joy to those we love can get intense.

Most of the time, we have a feeling that we are letting someone, or something important in our lives, down. We know we could or should be a better parent, partner, friend, daughter, son, sibling, employee, entrepreneur, artist, cook, or [insert what matters to you most].

The problem is that the world today is so loud and so busy, that it can all feel overwhelming.

It can feel overwhelmingly negative.

Sure, we've all read that optimists live longer, enjoy better health, and attract more friends and success. The problem is that when stress, anxiety, illness, or just pure bad-luck kick in, that extra dose of negative news or interaction with your boss can pitch you into negativity.

Just like joy vibrates outward and is contagious, so too is a dark mood and outlook. Get one person complaining bitterly and watch the conversation take a turn for the worst. The next time those around you are in a stressed out funk, try shaking them up a bit. Ask them about their favorite time of day, or the last time delight flooded out the noise of pressure and expectation.

## Step 5: Yoga Yourself

Why does yoga boost your self-esteem? You start to build an inner fire when you show up every day on your yoga mat. You will feel proud that you commit to practice and follow through, even if this commitment is just ten minutes per day.

With time you will master poses you never thought possible, achieve flexibility you only dreamed of, and gradually slim to a healthy weight. There will be a surge of confidence the first time you kick up into a handstand, or your heels touch the floor in downward dog. When you start a regular yoga practice you begin to show up for yourself by taking responsibility for your physical, mental, and perhaps spiritual wellness too. By engaging in self-respect, if not self-love, you will raise your self-esteem.

## Step 6: Give Dark Emotions Space to Be.

Yes, you read that correctly. First I told you to write out a joy-list, to add more of those experiences into your life, and to talk more about joy with everyone you meet.

Now I'm telling you to sit on the ground and do nothing. Yes, I mean literally.

Meditation is a way to open yourself up and to be more of yourself by feeling connected to everyone and everything. Meditation will unleash your joy in a way nothing else can. Sitting and watching your thoughts glide past as you focus on your breath will unleash some negative emotions. The noise and business of life can block out the anger, sadness, shame, and fear. All of those emotions can bubble up while you sit still, in silence. You may have been unaware they were just below the surface.

Do you know what is gorgeous about giving dark emotions space to surface? It may take weeks, or months, or years, but the fear will seep away. With time, the negative emotions will roll through you without invoking a knee-jerk reaction to smother them with food, entertainment, noise, achievement, work, or positive experiences. You will be able to allow anger, sadness, pain, and fear to flow in without losing your balance. You will be able to stop running and to stop grasping, knowing all things pass, and this, whatever it is, will move too.

## Step 7: Intensify the Positive

Have you seen a happy child jumping up and down with excitement at a holiday celebration? When small children learn to do something for the first time they throw their hands up in the air, or start do a happy dance, or begin to laugh. Children know how to intensify their positive emotions. We can learn from them how to open to more joy. From now on, when you reach a goal, have a lucky break, or are joyful at the sight of a sunrise, INTENSIFY the feeling by throwing your arms open, pumping your fist into the sky, doing a happy dance, jumping up and down a few times, or laughing out loud. If nothing else, do an internal happy dance.

*"When you are inspired by some great purpose, some extraordinary project, all your thoughts break their bonds; your mind transcends limitations; your conscious expands in every direction; and you find yourself in a great, new and wonderful world." Patanjali*

## TAKE ACTION:

Step 1: Write your daily, monthly, and year JOY-LISTS.

Step 2: Schedule JOY into your daily life, as well as mini-month joy-cations.

Step 3: Relate to people in a new way by asking and sharing sources of joy.

Step 4: Turn the conversation to sources of happiness instead of negativity, gossiping, or complaining.

Step 5: Yoga Time: Find a YouTube video or head to your local yoga studio.

Step 6: Meditate. You can start with just five minutes a day to make a difference.

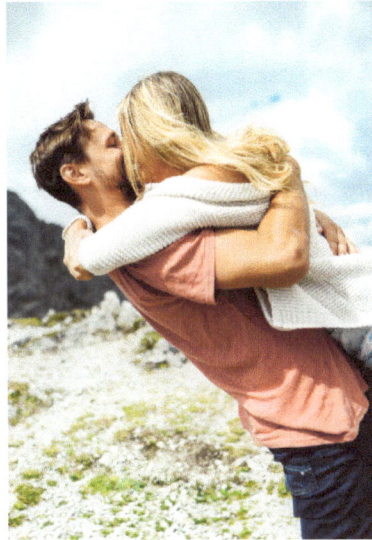

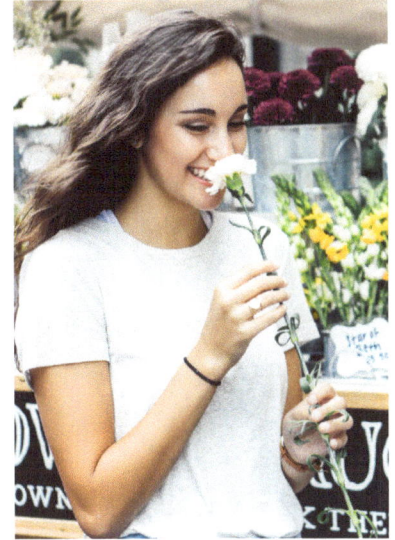

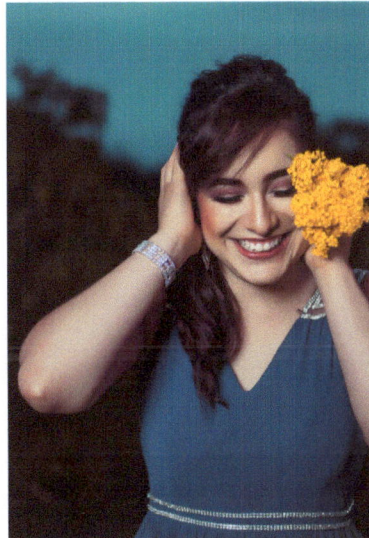

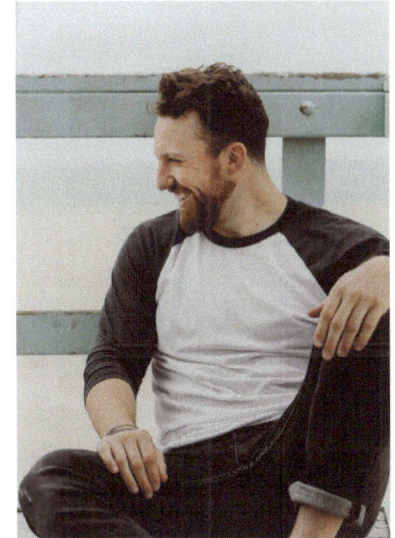

# Negative Emotions- How to Cope

What do you reach for or do when negative emotions, pain, or stress push you out of balance? If you reach for a cigarette every time you are stressed, don't judge yourself harshly. Your body is clever. You are reaching for a way to bring your body back into balance. And smoking, or eating sugar, or having a drama melt-down works in the short term. Unfortunately, unhealthy re-balancing mechanisms negatively impact your health, well-being, and joy within minutes, hours, days, or years. The answer is to create YOUR own list of healthy, positive, happiness-inducing activities to do INSTEAD of your current unhealthy re-balancing mechanism. You may think you don't need to write your well-being list down, but it is essential.

**WE CAN'T THINK CLEARLY** when we are in the grips of intense negative emotion or pain. You need a list of options you can turn to, or you will fall into the familiar groove you have created in your mind to reach for a smoke, a brownie, a glass of wine, or start a fight. In the end, love is the primary force in our lives. Most of our negative emotions come from a lack of love for ourselves and others. I don't know about you, but I struggle to keep my heart open when faced with mean-ness, rejection, hostility, or aggression.

When I feel less than, or fail, the stress response kicks in and I want to hide. What is your reaction? Do you want to fight? Do you freeze?

We can work to build our compassion and wrap ourselves and the situation in healing light. This can take just a few minutes of full mindfulness and the space of three deep breaths between trigger and response. Sometimes that means removing ourselves from the situation and nourishing ourselves with time in nature, yoga, meditation, appreciating beauty, exercising, taking a nap, easing into a bath, or asking for affection or support from someone loving. Build spaciousness around the negative feelings instead of wanting to run away, suppress, or cover them up. Allow the feelings to be while observing yourself and your thoughts. Last of all, don't judge and beat yourself up internally for falling out of balance and into negative emotions. Culture wants to define success as material wealth accumulation, fame, or being happy all the time. Perhaps we should be more concerned with how quickly we can reopen our heart while retaining our inner sense of self worth and balance. Kindness, patience, humility, creativity, devotion, passion, love.

## Negative Emotions: How to Cope Action Steps:

**STEP 1:** Take the time to create well-being and joy lists for yourself and carry them with you for reference. You can use my joy and well-being list ideas on the following pages for inspiration.

**STEP 2:** The next time negative emotions flood in, pushing you out of balance, PAUSE and take three deep breaths, making the exhale twice as long as the inhalation. Breathe in for three counts. Breathe out for six. Just be with the emotion. No matter how much you want to escape how you are feeling, be brave and sit still with how you are feeling for at least a few minutes. Try a yin yoga class if you need to do some healing work.

**STEP 3:** Look at your well-being and joy lists. Choose one activity to do to bring your body, mind, and soul back into balance that will promote both short and long-term health, wellness, and joy.

**STEP 4:** Accept the situation if there is nothing you can do and release negativity. Surrender. Otherwise take ACTION to improve the situation so that you can create enthusiasm, love, or contentment.

*"There is always a light within us that is free from all sorrow and grief, no matter how much we may be experiencing suffering." -Patanjali*

# Releasing Addictions

When you open to joy you will still have negative emotions show up. What do you do when negative emotions flood your system or sneak up on you? What is your go-to way to bring your body, mind, and feelings back to equilibrium?

*Between stimulus and response there is the chance to choose.*

Numbing thoughts and emotions are possible by escaping into television, video games, drugs, shopping, exercise, smoking, trying to control everything or everyone around you, seeking the pity of others, becoming a martyr and serving others at the sacrifice of personal well-being, and becoming a workaholic. Some people reach for a glass of wine or an entire bottle. Others reach for French fries, brownies, or other fat, sugar, and salty food. Still, others lash out at those around them or create drama to distract themselves from deep emotions and issues they don't want to face. Then there are those that can't or won't use any way to try to calm, heal, or uplift how they are feeling. They get into bed and stay there. Or they plaster a smile on their face and trudge forward with their life, just trying to get through another day.

There is a better way to cope with negative emotions. It isn't what happens to you, but your reaction to it; it is the sometimes split-second pause between stimulus and response that will change your life forever. Just as we can train our muscles to become stronger, so too can we train an inner spaciousness.

1. The next time you feel sadness, shame, anger, despair, rage, resentment, grief, hopelessness, fear, or any other negative emotion, pause.

2. Place one hand on your belly and one hand over your heart. If you can't do this in the current situation, then imagine your hands are resting there.

3. Take a deep breath in through the nose, filling first your belly, then your low ribs, feel your heart expand outward and upward. Exhale out the nose, allowing your shoulders to soften down your back body.

4. Breathe in three more times in this way if time permits. Count up to three on your inhalation, and down from six to one on your exhalation.

Breathing out twice as slowly as you inhale will allow the stress response in your body to turn off, and the healing parasympathetic system to turn on.

5. Now imagine floating above yourself in the third person. Just observe. Attach your mind to the breath. Inhale for three counts, exhale for six.

6. Grow still. Be with whatever emotions are here, or arising from moment to moment.

7. Imagine with each in-breath you are creating more inner space for the feelings to unclench and flow.

With each out breath feel yourself softening around whatever emotions are within you right now. You may feel an urge to run. Be brave. Stay still.

8. Name the emotion. Release all thoughts about the feeling. Accept whatever emotion is here, right now, without acting on it in any way. Just be still, be with whatever is right now.

9. From this place of quiet, inner spaciousness, decide what you can do, right now, at this moment, to

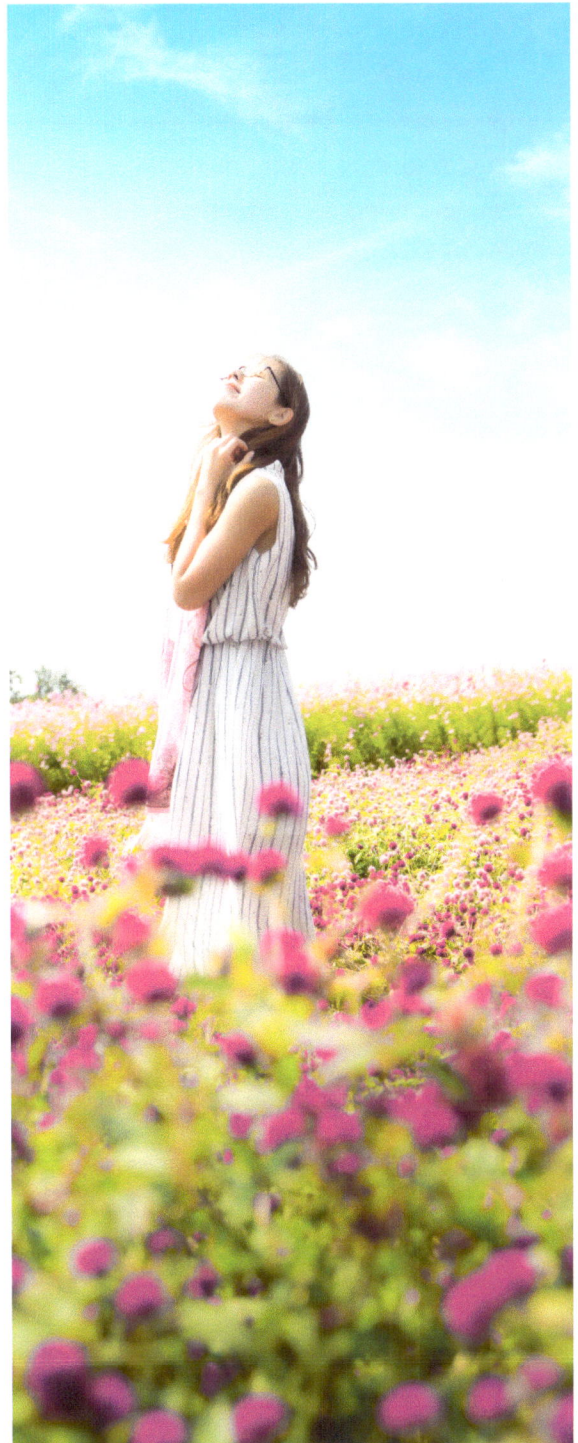

improve your situation. You can take out your joy and well-being lists. What can you do at this moment to nourish your body, mind, or soul to increase your well-being? If you can do nothing, then accept what is and release struggle. Release negativity. Attach your mind over and over again to the breath. Inhale for three, exhale for six. Cultivate your inner spaciousness for as long as you need, or as time permits. If you still feel the clutch of the negative emotions, then return to this exercise and flow back through the steps.

*"The moment you let go of some old habit or conditioning, the instant you catch yourself in a programmed reaction, the self shifts." -Deepak Chopra*

10. A Yin Yoga or Restorative Yoga class can open up space for you to flow through the above steps and be still with whatever emotions are within you. We store repressed trauma and feelings in our bodies. Yin yoga especially allows us to open up the body and release old emotions from our muscles, fascia, and tissues. Yin Yoga can also keep new feelings from building tension, tightness, or pain in the body.

*"Aversion is a form of bondage. We are tied to what we hate or fear. That is why, in our lives, the same problem, the same danger or difficulty, will present itself over and over again in various prospects, as long as we continue to resist or run away from it instead of examining it and solving it." Patanjali*

Be patient while training inner spaciousness. Continue through the steps, and you will eventually build inner strength. Your inner spaciousness will allow negative emotions to flow within you without you needing to grab a distraction or numbing mechanism, such as a plate of brownies.

Instead, you will become like a curious, loving, third-person observer. You will be strong enough to observe an emotion, name it, be with it, and the negative emotion will dissipate, like steam.

# Create Your Well-being List

1. **YOGA** is the number one go-to for you to re-balance your body, mind, emotions, and spirit. Stressed and frantic? Yoga will calm you. Depressed or sad? Yoga will lift your mood and energy. The effects of yoga last long after you get up off your yoga mat. Yoga will lower your baseline stress levels and relieve anxiety while boosting your daily well-being.

Perhaps you've heard about yoga. Your keen to try yoga after work. It's just that you're exhausted, the kids are hungry, and you're overwhelmed. You used up your willpower hours ago at work, and it's unavailable to pull you onto your yoga mat or to a yoga studio. What if I told you that after just 30 days, you could get your brain and body addicted to yoga, so won't need willpower?

You will start craving a yoga vinyasa flow session. Doubtful? Did you know that there is a positive correlation between practicing yoga and an increase in thalamic GABA levels in your brain? Scientists discovered in a clinical trial that yoga worked better than walking over 12 weeks to boost mood, well-being and to lower anxiety. The combination of breath work and movement in yoga increases GABA levels, which bind to receptors to produce an effect similar to how you feel after drinking a glass of wine. Unlike the glass of wine, the positive impact continues for

*"Asanas bring perfection in body, beauty in form, grace, strength, compactness, and the hardness and brilliance of a diamond."- Patanjali*

hours after a yoga session. Turn to yoga to bring yourself back to balance and well-being.

2. **Hug.** Throw those arms wide open and get ready to get and give eight hugs a day. Hugs release the hormone oxytocin, which functions as a neurotransmitter in the brain. Hold off on hugging it out with your arch rival or that energy vampire just yet. You'll experience a boost in mood and well-being if you hug and are hugged by someone you like and trust.

3. **Make New Friends, but Keep the Old.** My Grandma always said you only need one true friend to beautify your life, but look for new friends everywhere. Open up to making friends of different ages, backgrounds, professions, and beliefs. Whether you are an introvert or extrovert, spending time each week connecting will boost your well-being.

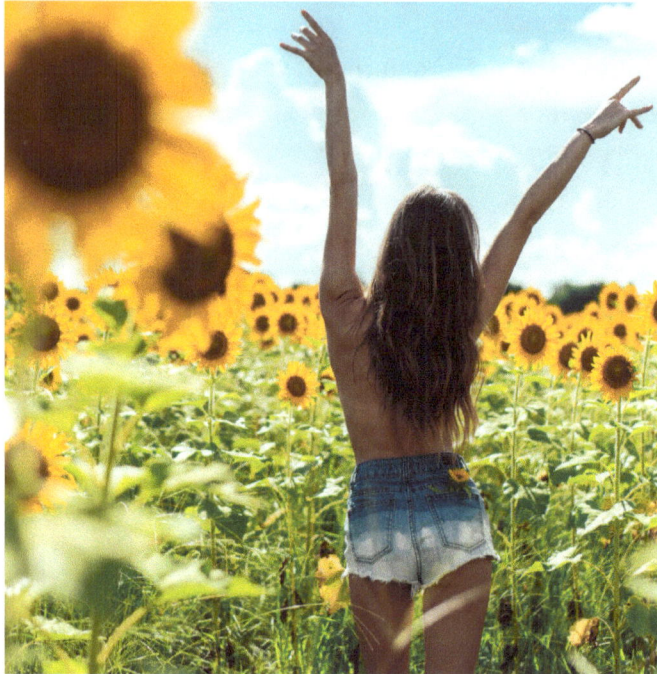

4. **Sun and Nature**. Ever notice how everyone is more cheerful on a sunny day? I'm sure it doesn't surprise you that studies correlate the amount of time spent outside with cheerfulness and positive emotions. Instinctively, we understand the power of the sun to infuse our lives with happiness. So why do most of us spend up to 90% of our lives inside? Walk outside during your morning break and over lunch time and let the power of the sun stimulate your serotonin production and boost your levels of vitamin D.

Making a conscious effort to step outside many times each day, even if it's just for one to two minutes at a time, can increase your well-being and lower your stress and anxiety. Invest in a sun lamp to mimic the natural sunlight in the winter months.

5. **Gifting releases dopamine in the brain**. So start giving gifts regularly to experience regular kicks of this feel-good chemical. You don't need to spend much to gain the benefits of giving. Gifting homemade presents such as bread, jams, homemade granola bars or treats, and personally created gift cards make beautiful presents. Gift time by volunteering.

6. **Laugh to skyrocket your well-being**. Go to a comedy show, turn on a laughter-inducing comedy show or movie or laugh with friends or family to release endorphins.

7. **Gratitude**. Write down a list of everything for which you are genuinely thankful. You will release serotonin in the brain and increase your well-being.

8. **Fast, Slow, Repeat.** Whether running, swimming laps in the pool, on a bike, or in a boat rowing, alternating bursts of sprinting and effort with slower paced recovery will ramp up your production of endorphins and give you a happy glow.

9. **Hydrotherapy.** A bath can melt stress for deep relaxation. Add drops of your favorite essential oil. Curl up with tea afterwards.

10. **OMMMMMM so Happy**. Meditation can increase your well-being and happiness. For best results for your happiness level, try twenty minutes each day.

11. **Go Minimal.** A bright, clean, but cozy space gives people a feeling of well-being. Try simplifying and de-cluttering your life to experience more happiness. Most people are unknowingly weighed down by their list of chores, clutter, and obligations.

Take out a garbage bag and toss out not only unloved or used items, but also resented or hated social obligations. Commit to a minimalist lifestyle to open up more space and freedom to fill with new experiences, beloved people, passions, and hobbies.

12. **Adrenaline Rush.** How much adrenaline does your unique brain need to feel well? If you are feeling fatigued or down, it could be that you are getting enough sleep, but not enough adventure.

Do something new, or try something outside your comfort zone. Try a ropes course, or go to a new meet-up or club.

13. **The Power of Touch to Uplift**. A massage and acupuncture increase the release of endorphins in the body. So go out for a massage, invest time in self-massage, or enjoy a massage from your love.

14. **Aromatherapy.** Spray some essential oil mist or use a diffuser to lift your mood, calm your

nervous system, or revitalize. Vanilla lowers anxiety, orange, lemon, and grapefruit uplift and energize, lavender calms, peppermint revitalizes, rosemary increases focus, and ylang-ylang soothes.

15. **Forest Bathing**. In a scientific study, researchers measured the effect of time spent in a forest on health and found that a day in the woods can lower stress, raise your energy level, lift your mood, boost your immune system, increase your sleep quality, and reduce recovery time from illness or surgery.

16. **Add Color**. Appreciating the beauty of fresh cut flowers on your desk, wearing a bright colored outfit, looking at a splash of color against white space, or rejoicing in the vivid colors of the meals on your plate at dinner can increase your well-being.

17. **Give it Up to Spice it Up.** Try giving up one of your standard activities to open up space for something new. Give up television, gaming, social media, crafting or shopping. Try new activities. Give yourself permission to look silly or fail.

Trying new things is exciting and tiring. Reward yourself with extra sleep.

18. **Be Sensual.** Whether you are in a relationship or not, open up space and time to be sensual to boost your well-being. Enjoy how good touch feels. Wear clothes that feel soft, smooth and cool, or cuddle against your skin. Go a day without wearing a bra. Try sleeping in the nude to appreciate how the sheets feel against your bare skin. Go skinny dipping in a pool or a lake. Experience the feel of the sun and the wind on your skin.

19. **Sleep** is a essential ingredient for well-being. Get eight hours of sleep a night. Nap to refresh.

20. Do you have a **Sense of Purpose**? Once our basic needs are met, we all need to feel that our lives matter. If you don't have a sense of purpose, then get into action and try new ways to make a difference. Then take time to feel into your inner being, pray, or meditate. Does this feel right?

Be patient and keep trying new ways to contribute. Give your ego a holiday when finding your sense of purpose. Your purpose may be helping orphans in poverty, or it could be bringing laughter and love to your workplace. It could be to inspire millions to use solar panels or care for a sick parent. Your purpose may not be what pays your bills.

21. **Imagine** you have the ideal life you want, right now. What do your relationships look like? What work do you do? How do you spend your time? How do you interact with people? Where do you live? Don't just dream it, but feel the positive emotions. Intensify them. Then take pen to paper and work backward and set goals. Break down the goals into steps and actions on a year, month, week, and daily level. List out the activities you'll need to do each day to reach your goals. Each time you meet your daily, weekly, and monthly goals celebrate with a mini-reward celebration, which will give you a kick of dopamine. Dopamine is our feel-good motivation fuel. Small, regular kicks of dopamine can give you the energy and positive reinforcement to continue.

Above all, release attachment to the end goal and the result of your efforts. Take a break a few times a day to feel gratitude flow through you for all the blessings in your life right now. The combination of action, gratitude, and release of attachment to a particular outcome will open up new opportunities. You may not even end up at the point you were aiming, but at a place far better than you could have ever imagined.

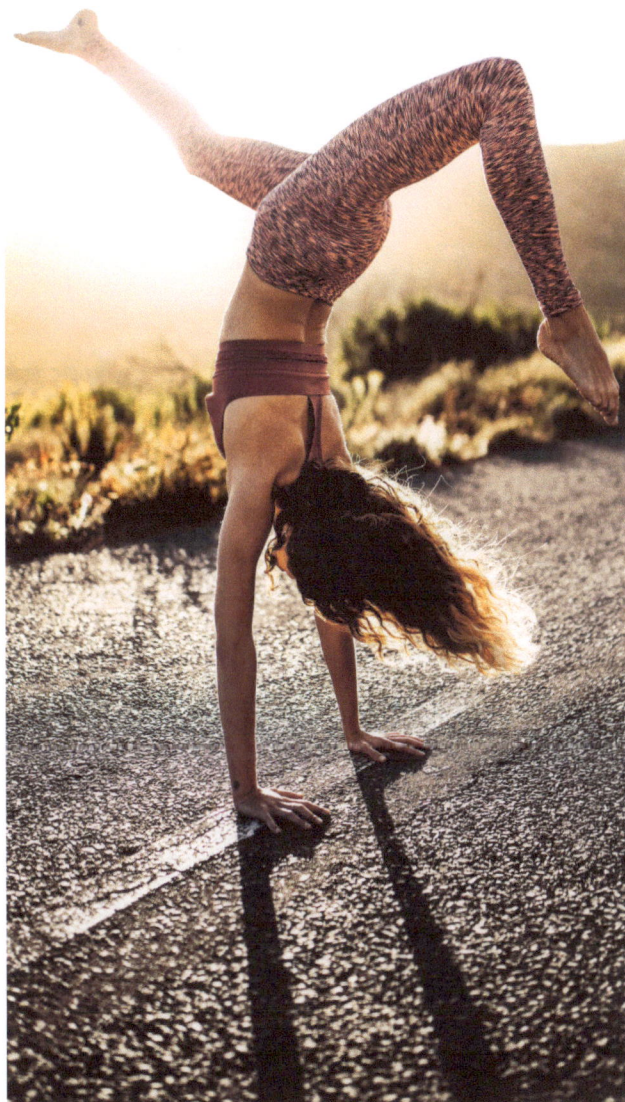

# Social Wellness Evaluation / Affirmations

| | Highly disagree | Disagree | Slightly disagree | Slightly agree | Agree | Strongly agree |
|---|---|---|---|---|---|---|
| • I have a loving relationship with myself. | | | | | | |
| • My internal voice is loving and supportive. | | | | | | |
| • If I am single, I am content with my status. | | | | | | |

If I am in a romantic relationship:

| | Highly disagree | Disagree | Slightly disagree | Slightly agree | Agree | Strongly agree |
|---|---|---|---|---|---|---|
| • I have a wonderful relationship with my partner. | | | | | | |
| • My relationship is quite romantic. | | | | | | |
| • We set aside plenty of time to spend alone together. | | | | | | |
| • Our sex life is very satisfying. | | | | | | |
| • We are affectionate: cuddling, hugging, kissing, daily. | | | | | | |
| • I know my partner's love language and act to speak it. | | | | | | |
| • My relationship with my partner feels exciting. | | | | | | |
| • My partner and I can communicate easily, honestly, and openly with each other. | | | | | | |
| • My love relationship is rarely a source of stress for me. | | | | | | |
| • I believe I am a very good partner and give the appropriate amount of energy to the relationship. | | | | | | |
| • I have taken time to reflect and know what kind of a relationship I want to be building. | | | | | | |
| • I have a satisfying, active social life. | | | | | | |
| • I have friends I can always count on to be there for me. | | | | | | |
| • I devote energy and time into my friendships. | | | | | | |

| | Highly disagree | Disagree | Slightly disagree | Slightly agree | Agree | Strongly agree |
|---|---|---|---|---|---|---|
| I give my time and energy to relationships that nourish versus the relationships that drain me. | | | | | | |
| I consider myself to be a very good friend. | | | | | | |
| I have thought deeply about my social wellness and know exactly what kind of friendships I want to build. | | | | | | |
| I have a close, loving relationship with my dad. | | | | | | |
| I have a close, loving relationship with my mom. | | | | | | |
| Overall, I have a close, loving relationship with my siblings and they can count on me to be there for them. | | | | | | |
| I have a loving close relationship with grandparents, aunts, uncles, or self-created family members. (Our birth family is not the only chance to build a family.) | | | | | | |
| I do something loving for my friends, family members or neighbors at least once a week. | | | | | | |

If I have children:

| | Highly disagree | Disagree | Slightly disagree | Slightly agree | Agree | Strongly agree |
|---|---|---|---|---|---|---|
| I have a close, loving, healthy relationship with my kids. | | | | | | |
| My parent strategy is conscious, and clearly defined. | | | | | | |
| I give each of my children individual, quality time every week. | | | | | | |
| I seldom experience anxiety with regard to my children. | | | | | | |
| My relationship with my kids is a source of joy. | | | | | | |
| I am setting a wonderful example for my children of how to live a beautiful life. | | | | | | |
| I am happy with the character and values of my kids. | | | | | | |
| Overall, I feel like I am an amazing parent. | | | | | | |

# Loving

The entire chapter on love is written for myself as a golden standard of how I want to show up in the world and in my relationships. Feel free to take any inspiration you may find in my love goals and create your own. What does a loving life of joy and well-being look like for you? How do you want to love?

## CONNECTING WITH LOVE

Acting from a place of love is less arduous when you are infused with well-being and serenity. Responding with love is a challenge when we are exhausted, in pain, stressed, or pushed to the limit. Thus most of us stand in awe of those who can act from a place of love despite intense pain or hardship.

The first step to connecting with more love is caring for our wellness by moving our bodies throughout the day, fueling our body with high-quality food and drink, and getting enough rest and sleep. Investing in steps to infuse more health and well-being into our lives sets us up to more easily act from a place of love.

> "Love is the master key that opens the gates of happiness."
> – Oliver Wendell Holmes

## LOVING WITHOUT CONDITION

Loving without clutching, controlling, retreating, jealousy, or fear is a challenge. So many relationships are built on the level of ego in an unspoken quid pro quo balance. Do you recognize yourself in any of the following attitudes to loving: I do this for you, and I expect you to do this for me. If you complete x,y,z, and behave in a certain way, then I like and love you, if you don't, then

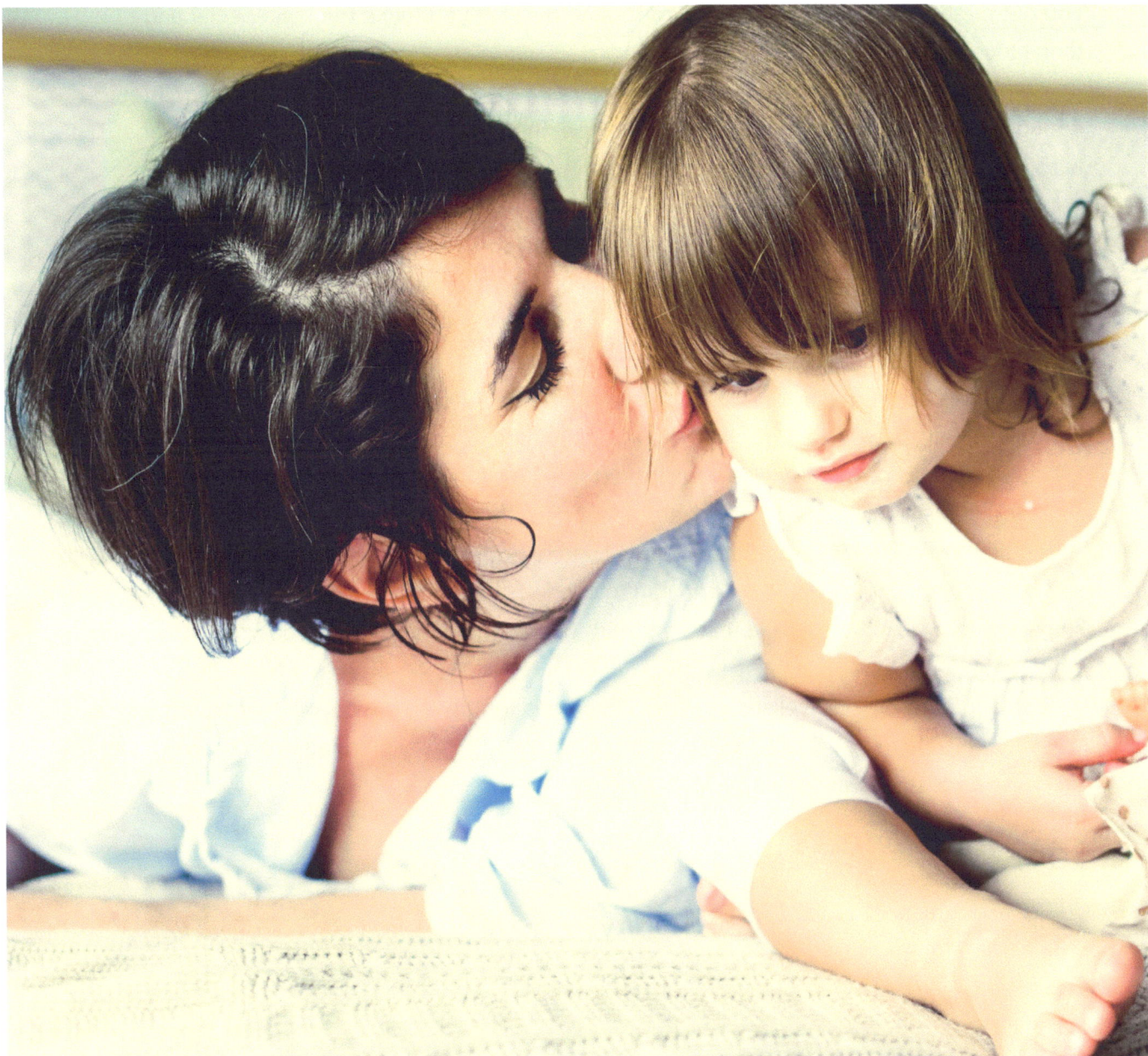

"Much depends on your attitude. If you are filled with negative judgment and anger, then you will feel separate from other people. You will feel lonely. But if you have an open heart and are filled with trust and friendship, even if you are physically alone, even living a hermit's life, you will never feel lonely." ~ Dalai Lama you get negative emotions from me or a turning away. If you make me feel special and unique, then I love you.

I need you to reassure me, over and over again, in different ways, and then I will feel safe enough to love you back. If you are THIS person, then I will love you. You must do things, THIS way, for me to like you. OR, I will do everything you ask, anything, just love me. I will bend over backward, love me, I need your love.

Loving without clutching, controlling, retreating, jealousy, or fear is possible when you open the flow of love and fill yourself up with love before opening the heart to others.

Love without conditions is something we yearn for on a deep level. Most of us seek this love outside of ourselves instead of on cultivating self-love, first. "Love yourself," is advice almost everyone has heard or read. But what does this mean? And could too much self-love be a bad thing? After all, doesn't it seem like there is a rising tide of narcissistic people everywhere?

Classic symptoms of narcissism are a need for excessive admiration, inability to accept criticism and obsession with perfection. Narcissistic people have even lower real self-love than most.

True self-love flows out of the heart center and is both self-sufficient and unconditional. With self-love you no longer require the admiration of others, power, fame, fortune, beauty, or relationships to feel whole. You love yourself without these conditions. So how do you cultivate more self-love?

By taking care of your wellness through the steps in this book, you will be igniting self-love. You can cultivate more self-love and love for others through daily meditation and coming into the present moment over and over again in your daily life.

## LOVE WITH EQUANIMITY MEDITATION

*"Be happy for those who are happy, have compassion towards the unhappy, and maintain equanimity towards the wicked." Patanjali Yoga Sutras*

Sit with a straight spine on a chair or cross-legged on the floor. Begin to deepen your breath. Place one hand on your belly, and the other on your heart. Inhale, feeling the breath expand into your belly, your low ribs, and lifting your heart towards the sky. Exhale and experience your heart descending, your shoulders relaxing down your back, your low back softening.

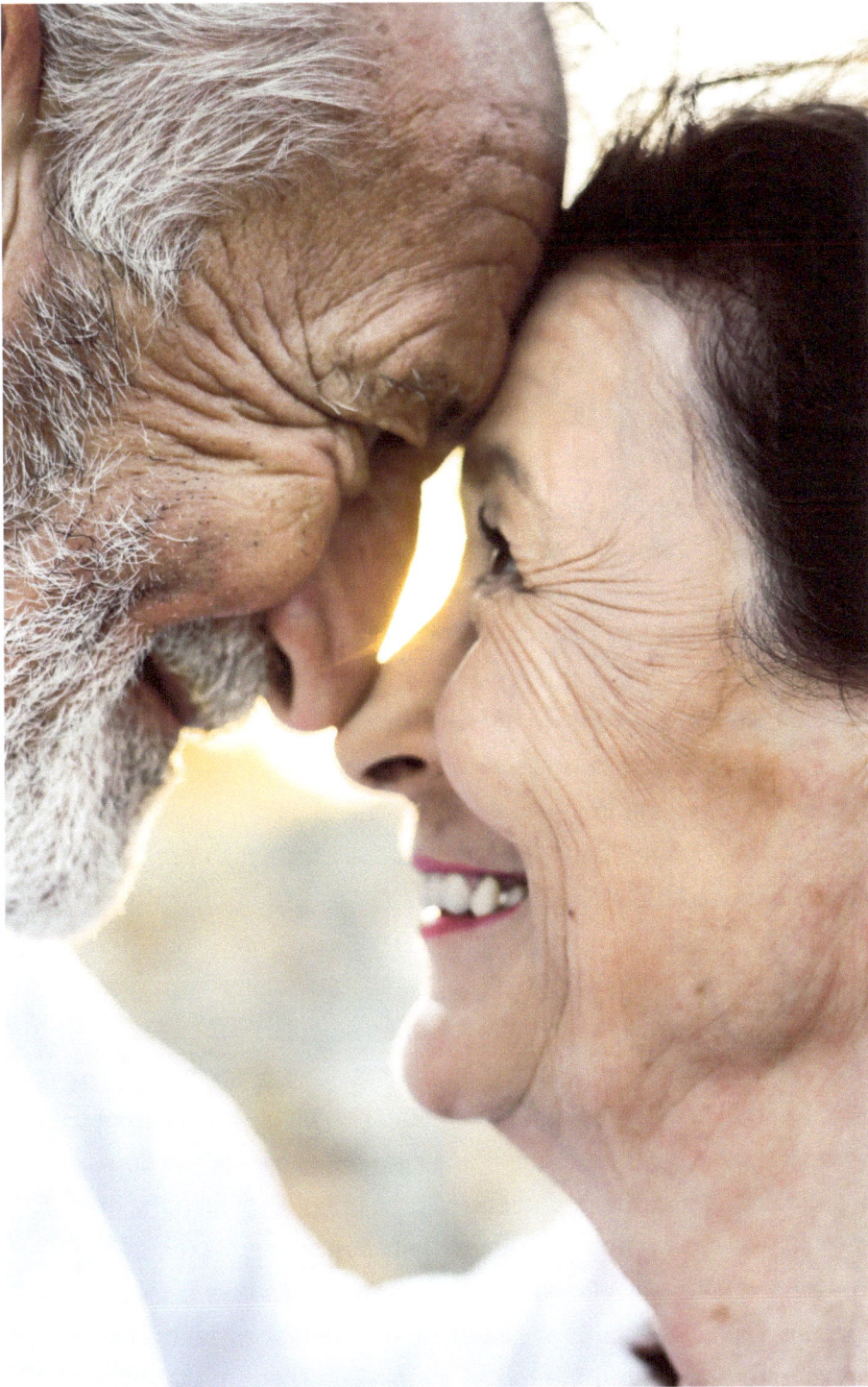
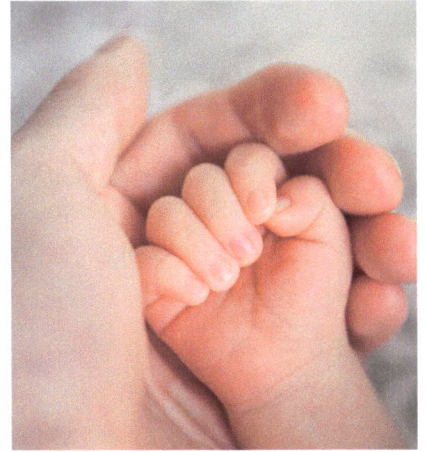
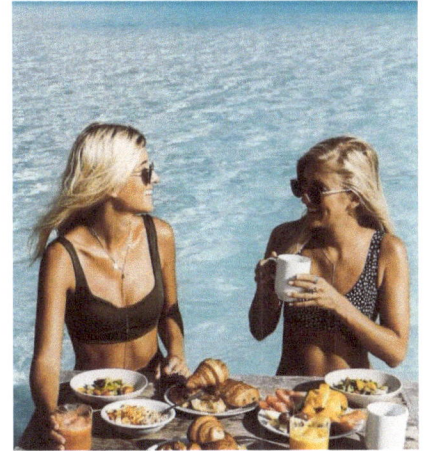
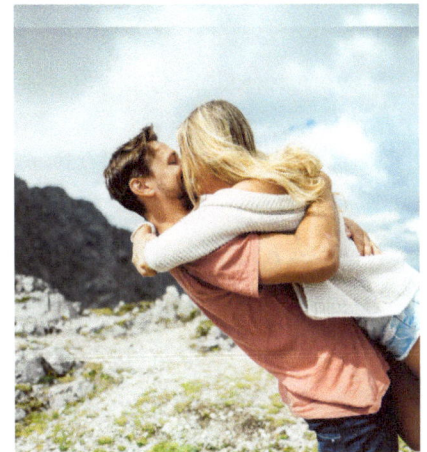

Breathe here for a few breaths, observing the breath in this flow. Next, place your left hand on your heart and your right hand on top of the left. Imagine a warm glow building in your heart center. Then bring your elbows to your sides and lift your hands, palm up, towards the sky, as if you are holding up a platter on your hands. Imagine love from your heart flowing out onto your hands. You are offering this love out to the world.

Now picture people walking by in front of you. People you love. People you like. People you dislike. People you don't know. See someone you love stop in front of you and scoop the love off your hands and press it to their heart. Watch their face light up with joy. How do you feel? Observe how you react in your body, heart, mind, and soul. Now see someone you like stop in front of you and consider the love offered on your palms. They tilt their head to the side, thinking for a moment, and then turn away from you and continue walking. They do not want your love, at least at this moment. How do you feel? Observe how you react in your body, heart, mind, and soul.

A stranger sees you out of the corner of their eye and pause, mid-step. They walk forward, and pause, hesitant. Gently, they sweep some of the love off your hands, holding it tentatively in their own palms. They look down at it, up at you, then back down. A soft smile light up their face. Their eyes flicker up to yours and then they continue walking. You see them passing people up along the road, the love still held in front of them in the palms of their hands. Many don't react. But one lifts the palms of their hands, and the love bounces onto their palms, and they smile.

Someone you dislike stops in front of you, regarding the love in your hands. How do you feel? Observe how you react in your body, heart, mind, and soul. Do you want to press your hands back to your heart? Is it an effort to keep your hands held out open?

Don't judge. Just watch your reaction. Next, they take a step forward, scoop the love out of your hands and stomp on it. Negative energy radiates toward you, hurling up against you. Watch your reaction. Can you keep your hands open? Can you retain an inner, steadfast serenity?

Now picture once again people walking by in front of you. People you love. People you like. People you dislike. People you don't know. See someone you love stop in front of you and scoop the love off your hands and press it to their heart. Watch their face light up with joy. How do you feel? Observe how you react in your body, heart, mind, and soul. Some people will take the love you offer. Some people will not. Not everyone needs to like you, and that's okay. You can feel your heart staying open, and it feels good. You feel relaxed. Deeper and deeper relaxed. Your entire body, every muscle, softens, releases any tension, relaxes, deeper and deeper. Take a deep breath in, and let it out. Imagine you are standing at the top of a stairway. There are ten steps down to a beautiful, safe place, perhaps somewhere in nature you've visited, or imagine. Take a deep breath in, and step onto the top stair.

Ten, step down, nine, take a deep breath in, and let it out as you step down, 9, going deeper and deeper. 8, 7, 6, feeling deeper relaxed with every step, 5, 4, 3, 2, 1. You step into your beautiful space and sit down, with your hands held out, palms up, in front of your heart. Feel warm golden energy flowing out of your heart center, onto your palms, and then rushing back over your entire body. Perhaps the golden energy flows back into your heart, sweeping like a wave from your heart out to every inch of your body. Maybe the golden energy bounces up to the crown of your head and washes down over every part of you to the tips of your toes.

Rest here, feeling the golden energy flow out of your heart, on to your palms, and back through your body. Press your left hand to your heart now, and the right hand over the left. Imagine your heart center flooding with an infinite supply of love for yourself for those you love, like, don't know, or dislike. Envision yourself in daily life, not pushing this love out, but offering this love upon the palms of your hands. People can take it, walk by, or hurl negative energy at you in response. It's all okay. You feel relaxed, and it's fine. Feel an equanimity building within you, an inner strength, a serenity. Count to ten now, and when you arrive at ten, you will open your eyes, feeling revitalized and full of love, 1, 2, 3, 4, 5, 6, 7, 8, 9, 10. Open your eyes. Wiggle your fingers and toes, and bow forward, touching your hands to the floor, grounding your energy. Rise up, smile, and return to your day.

## THE POWER & ART OF APOLOGIZING

Few people can apologize well. Employing an authentic, sincere, and brave apology is powerful. So how can you do this well?

1. Validate their feelings so they feel understood.
2. Make a statement regretting what you have done.
3. Say you are sorry with sincerity and that you will effort for it to never happen again.
4. ESSENTIAL INGREDIENT: Ask for forgiveness and be patient. Sometimes they need time.
5. In some situations, look for how you can make amends for the damage you caused.

## LOVING PROBLEM RESOLUTION

We all have desires, and that's okay. Desire propels us forward in life to learn, grow, love, and experience the richness of life. Conflict can spark when the desire of two or more people contradict. Then the conflict just needs a splash of shame, guilt, manipulation, or fear for a fire of trouble to ignite. Here is an example. Your mother wants your family to come to spend Christmas with her. There is nothing wrong with this desire. Nor is there anything wrong with you wanting to celebrate Christmas at home. The conflict takes flame when guilt and manipulation are thrown on the kindling. So often this happens in relationships. I want what I desire, but I also want you to want it, too. If you say you don't want what I wish or want something different, then I can use shame, guilt, manipulation, a retracting of affection or love, or even fear to make you ACT like you've changed your mind.

You go along, put on a smile, and pretend you want what I desire. You push resentment and anger down, where it simmers. Or you let it go because you tell yourself you are an easy going person, and you didn't care, anyway.

What is a loving problem resolution method? How do we stop employing shame, guilt, manipulation, a retracting of affection or love, or even fear to stimulate people to do what we want? The answer is compassion, empathy, and brave honesty. Speak up. Say what you desire. Insist other people say what they want using I statements, instead of sentences beginning with "we," or "we should," or "you." Every once in a while, it could be that everyone genuinely wants the same thing.

Much more often desires contradict. The answer is never to compromise. Compromise means no one gets what they want and everyone is at least a touch disappointed or resentful. Either one person gets their way, someone else does, or a new synergy third option is created that both love. If one person gets their way, then they need to thank the oth-

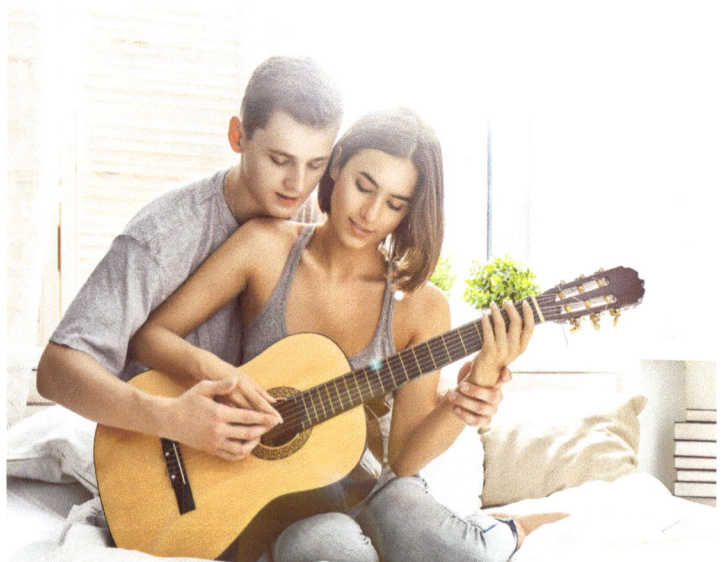

34

ers, who say, "you're welcome". There is no pretending needed. You would be surprised how effective it is to state, succinctly, what you want and be ready to accept a no. Here is a quick example: "I would like us to go to brunch with my parents every Sunday morning. Are you willing to do that for me?"

"I would prefer to sleep late on Sunday, but yes, I'm willing to do it for you."

"Thank you."

*"Your task is not to seek for love, but merely to seek and find all the barriers within yourself that you have built against it." – Rumi*

## LOVING, HIGH QUALITY NO

What if, no matter how hard you try, someone refuses to lay down the shaming, guilting, manipulation, and games. What if they refuse to openly state what they want and that they will be grateful for you to help them fulfill their desire?

It is time to employ the loving, high quality no described by Eckhart Tolle. Such moments are a perfect time to practice saying no, firmly and resolutely, without any attached negative feelings. You don't need to give explanations, reasoning, or excuses. You can say no. No, I don't want to do that. No, that doesn't work for me. No, that is not going to happen. Say no without anger, resentment, or fear. Smile, and imagine your heart center opening up and staying open as you say no. Saying no, calmly, without explanation, with love, is a challenge. Be brave.

On the flip side, cultivate an ability to take no for an answer. Place yourself into the other person's shoes. What does it feel like to be looking out at this situation through their eyes? Then take a third person perspective, like a journalist or someone hovering above the room. Next, ask open-ended questions to find out more about why they don't want to say yes. Work hard to understand any of their fears or desires that contradict with what you want. Through dialogue, you could come to an even better, synergistic new solution, or you will understand the no, and the person, better. Begin to declare what you want, and ask others to help you get what you desire. Encourage others to do the same. Be willing to take turns.

Sometimes it will be time to lay down what you want, to comply with someone else's wishes.

Saying, "I am happy to do this for you," without calculating a quid pro quo in your mind, will feel like a taking a drink of your favorite hot beverage on a cold day. Loving without condition will warm you from the inside.

*"If there is no joy or happiness at the mental level, too much worrying, too much fear, then even the physical comforts and pleasure will not soothe your mental discomfort. Develop a genuine sense of love and affection." ~ Dalai Lama*

## DRAMA & ADDICTION RELEASE

Are you addicted to drama? How much drama is there in your life?

Even if you aren't initiating the drama, your energy could be drawing it to you. You may not be conscious of your craving for drama. You may think you hate the emotional roller coaster, conflict, and pain. You could be addicted to the associated adrenaline rush, the attention, and excitement. There is a reason why people find soap operas and tabloids entertaining. Drama gives the mind and the ego something on which to focus.

Around and around the thoughts swirl around the conflict, memory, situation. Drama gives you a story to tell and elicits attention. Or it could be that you use drama, unconsciously, as a distraction or excuse not to look at deep problems. You aren't living your best life, the life your soul wants you to live. Or there is so much pain that you want a distraction, even if that distraction layers on more pain. Society doesn't shame drama addicts the way it does binge eaters, alcoholics, smokers, or drug abusers. The principle, however, is the same.

One is using something to escape what is, at this moment. It could be as banal as boredom, unease, internal agitation. Or it could be anywhere on the bandwidth to the horrific, such as excruciating pain, either physical, mental, emotional, social, or spiritual. So what is the solution to stopping an addiction? First, lay down judgment. Recognize that when you reach for whatever it is you are addicted, you are seeking to bring your body, mind, emotions, or spirit into balance again. We all long to escape pain and desire happiness. There is nothing wrong with the martini or the pizza in and of itself. You were using whatever it is as a means of achieving equilibrium again. The problem is that it is only a short term solution. When the martini wears off, or the pizza is gone, the imbalance and negative feelings quickly return. So a cycle begins, and perhaps you need more, and more, to achieve balance. You need new go-to solutions to achieve balance. It is difficult to think clearly when we are stressed, in pain, anxious, exhausted, sad, angry, lonely, or feeling awful inside. Brainstorm a list of alternate options you can reach for to bring balance back into your body, mind, emotions, and soul. Write the list down, and keep it handy. The next time you want to reach for a cigarette, pizza, martini, creating drama, or whatever the go-to is for you that you want to stop, PAUSE. Take a deep breath in through the nose as you sweep the arms up to the sky. Exhale out the mouth as you fold forward over your legs. Grab opposite elbows, and hang here, with slightly bent knees, breathing deeply. Bring your attention to your feet, up your legs, hips, torso, arms, shoulders, neck, to the crown of your head. Feel into your body.

Next, bring your attention to whatever you are feeling. Release judgment. Directly observe what you are feeling. Make space for the emotions. Allow whatever arises to flow up. If your mind begins to churn with thoughts, watch them. If tears roll down your cheeks, permit the release. Reground into your body by bringing your awareness from the tips of your toes, up each part of your body, to the top of your head, and down again. After a few deep breaths, slowly stand back up, bring your hands to your heart.

Ask yourself where you need balance. For example, you could feel wired, but tired. You want to calm down, and relax, but are too tired to exercise, or do anything.

Reach for your list of healthy ideas.

One option is to lay flat on the floor for ten to twenty moments, with one hand on your chest and the other on your heart. Breathe deeply, feeling first your hand on your belly lift, then the hand over your heart. Or you could turn on your favorite music and dance, take a bath, or select a relaxing meditation visualization, or stress-relief hypnotherapy session. If you only have a few minutes, opt to lay down, flat on the floor and breathe deeply. You may be able to break your addiction in a moment. Most likely it will take time. Do not get discouraged. Just keep bringing presence into what you are feeling. Run through the steps in the exercise over and over again. Become a detective, searching out the why. Seek to solve the imbalance in new, healthy ways with your list of options. Dive deep, seeking to find healing instead of patching up the hole with short term fixes. Meditate daily. Try yin yoga. Spend time in nature. Get in touch with your soul. Angels are everywhere. You can ask them to help you. And you may find one day you are sitting in the sun, enjoying a martini, not because you need it, but because it is fun. Someone could snatch it out of your hands after the first sip, and you would shrug. You don't need it.

## LOVING KINDNESS

What one person loves and appreciates, another is indifferent about or hates. As you begin to encourage others to state openly what they desire, you will learn what you can do to surprise them with acts of loving kindness. Most people have one particular way that causes them to feel loved. It may be through presents, quality time spent together, physical affection, acts of service, or words of praise, gratitude, or support.

What makes the people in your life feel loved more than anything else? Is it a bunch of flowers? A hug? Someone surprising you with a clean house when you get home, or a home cooked meal? Is it a thoughtfully written card of support? Compliments? An afternoon spent together talking? If you aren't sure, ask them.

Begin to schedule in one surprise act of loving kindness per day. Watch how not only your relationships, but your life changes.

*"If you develop a strong sense of concern for the well-being of sentient beings and in particular all human beings, this will make you happy in the mornings, even before coffee." ~ Dalai Lama*

## LOVING PRESENCE

Almost everyone wants a safe place to find rest. Someone to listen to challenges or heartache, to lift us when we're down, open up arms to fall into when we need comfort. You may think that you need to solve the problems of those you love, but you don't. You don't need to be able to give good advice or distract them from their pain with alcohol, gifts, food, or laughter. You can be. Cultivate a loving presence of serenity and open your heart and ears. It is easier said than done. Few can tolerate holding space for dark emotions. Therefore we judge or seek to fix, cover, up, ignore, or run away from people with these emotions. Being a loving presence means you don't need to agree or validate. Just listen and allow any emotions that come forth from the person in front of you to flow out. Be with the person in front of you with all of your awareness, open your heart, and cultivate a spaciousness inside, a stillness, a settling into right now.

"The meaning of life always changes, but it never ceases to be. We can discover meaning in life in three different ways: (1) by creating a work or doing a deed; (2) by experiencing something – such as goodness, truth and beauty – by experiencing nature or culture or, by experiencing another human being in his very uniqueness – by loving him; and (3) by the attitude we take toward unavoidable suffering. Even the helpless victim of a hopeless situation, facing a fate he cannot change, may rise above himself, may grow beyond himself, and by so doing change himself."

Viktor E. Frankl

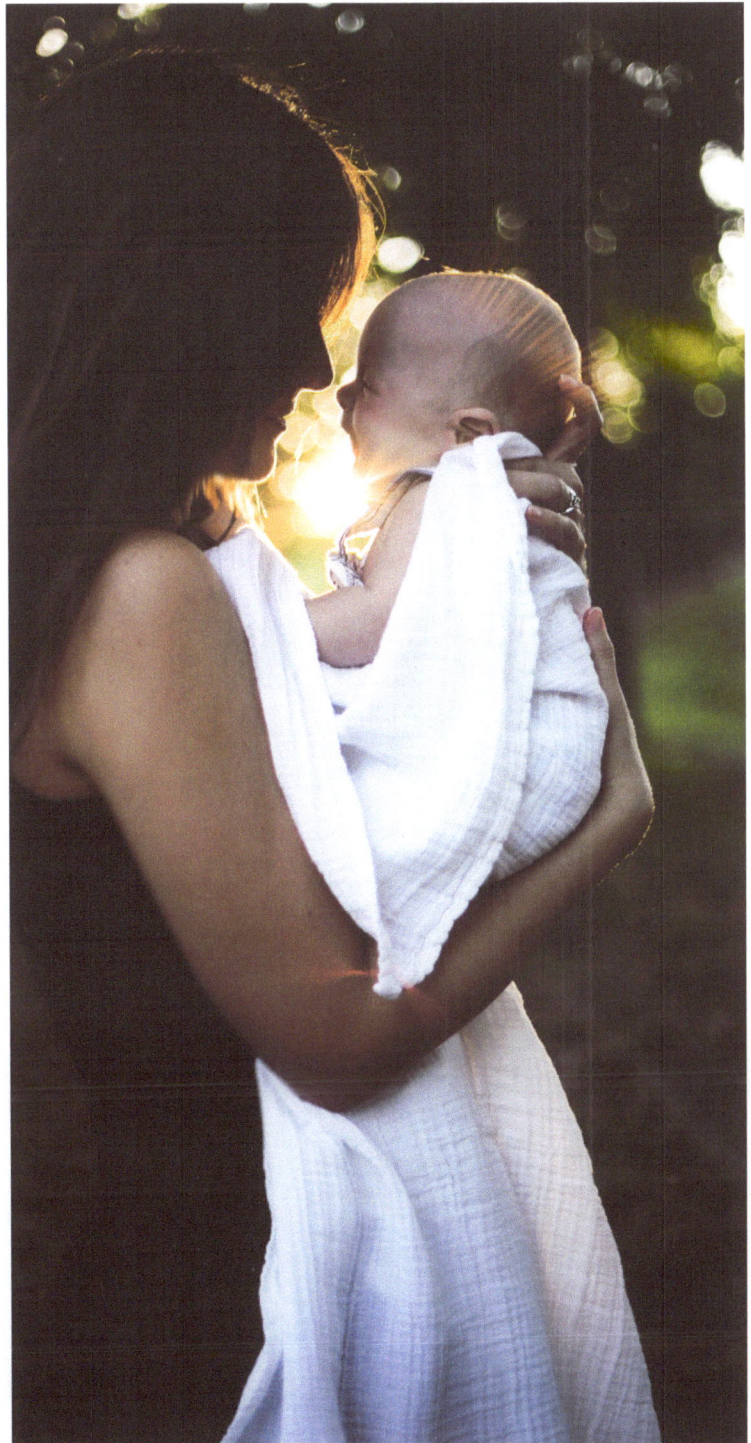

39

# WHAT ARE THE HABITS OF HAPPY COUPLES?

**LOVE HABIT # 1**
## BRAVE IT

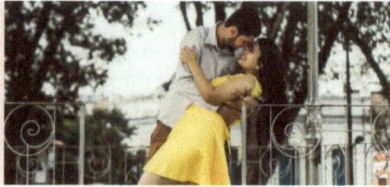

**Blissful couples aren't afraid....**To be the one who loves more, gives more, or forgives the fastest.

**LOVE HABIT # 2**
## FIGHT WITH LOVE

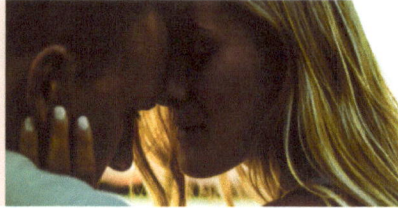

**Are you fighting with kindness & love?**
Healthy couples disagree. The question is how you fight. Happy couples don't yell, call names, say things to injure one another, give the silent treatment, or avoid each other. Instead, they listen, try to understand and take the time to work through problems and disagreements.

**LOVE HABIT # 3**
## APOLOGIZE & FORGIVE

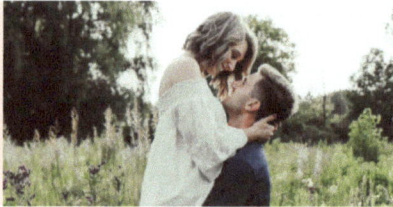

**Can you ASK for forgiveness?** And can you GIVE forgiveness? One secret of happy couples is that they make a habit of acknowledging they made a mistake and asking for forgiveness. They take action to make reparations. Happy couples forgive faster, trusting an apology is real.

**LOVE HABIT # 4**
## TRUST

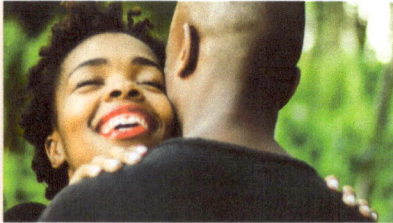

**Home is in your arms....**
Happy couples create safety and cozy security for each other. They become for one another truly 'home' and a safe place to fall. Really listening to each other builds security. Seeing and accepting your love for who they are, instead of who you want them to be, is the foundation.

**LOVE HABIT # 5**
## PATIENCE

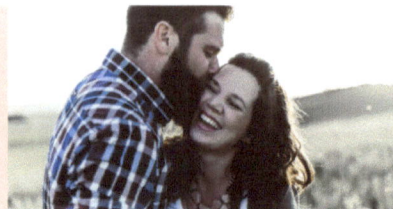

**WAIT.... You're NOT perfect?**
The strong will fall, the patient will lash out, the trustworthy will break a promise, and the organized will lose their keys...Blissful couples elevate each other to try to be the best version of themselves while holding their arms open wide for when each other fail.

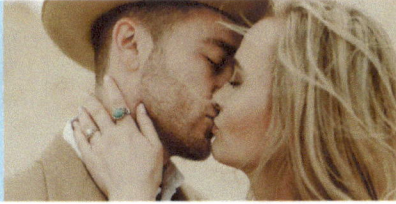

**LOVE HABIT # 6**
# KISS

**LOVE HABIT # 7**
# ADORE

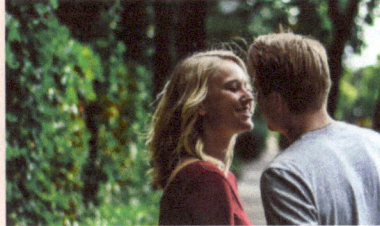

**LOVE HABIT # 8**
# COMPLIMENT

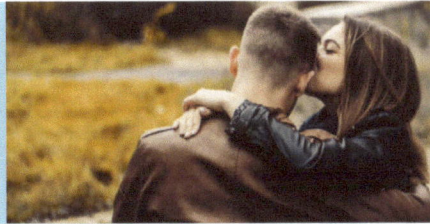

**LOVE HABIT # 9**
# USE HUMOR

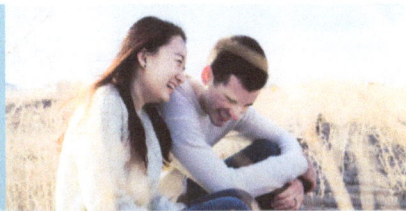

**LOVE HABIT # 10**
# TOUCH

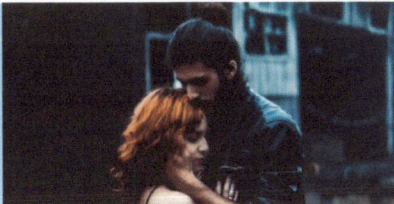

**Do you kiss goodbye and hello everyday?**
It can get easy to forget to kiss or hug hello and goodbye. Happy couples make a conscious decision to send their partner out the door and bring them home with a kiss.

**How do you talk about your partner?**
When you fall in love you can't stop thinking - or perhaps talking - about all the reasons your partner is marvelous. Hey, it's normal that your partner no longer dominates your thoughts after the first rush. But happy couples focus on what they love and admire, instead of what annoys them. They talk about why they adore their LOVE with friends and family instead of complaining.

**Do you compliment each other daily?**
Happy couples compliment each other and build each other up regularly. They offer up positive, supporting, and encouraging words of affirmation daily.

**Humor to laugh, defuse, & connect.**
Laughter releases endorphins in the brain. Couples that laugh together can associate each other with regular doses of feel-good chemicals. A secret habit of happy couples is their use of humor in a fight. Happy couples use humor to defuse a fight.

**Hold hands, hug, kiss, and massage....**
Want to know a secret of happy couples? They touch often. They hold hands, give each other foot or shoulder massages, hug, and give a loving pat as they walk by. You can trigger oxytocin while lowering blood pressure and cortisol levels by just hugging your partner for 25 seconds.

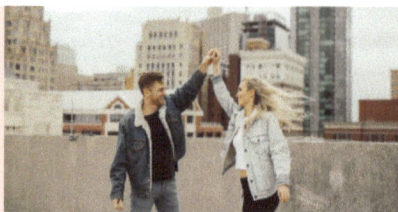

**LOVE HABIT # 11**

## ONE TEAM

### Keeping score...

Is not a habit of happy couples. They both pitch in to build and maintain a life together. Beyond that, they find little acts of service they can do to lighten their partner's work or inspire a smile.

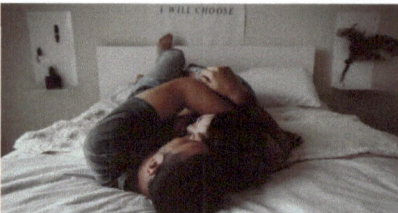

**LOVE HABIT # 12**

## SEX & MONEY

### Let's talk about sex...

And about our finances. Happy couples take the plunge and discuss money and about what they need in forms of intimacy in the bedroom. Being on the same wavelength about how to spend and how to satisfy fortifies a relationship.

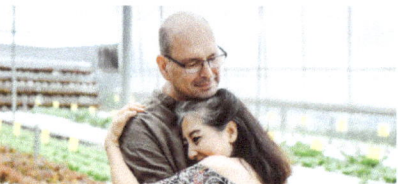

**LOVE HABIT # 13**

## GRATITUDE

### Why does a thank you mean so much?

Happy couples have a secret weapon against resentment; they thank each other regularly for both big and little things they do.

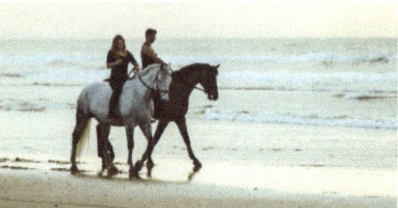

**LOVE HABIT # 14**

## TALK & WALK

### Even with hectic schedules and stress...

Happy couples make it a habit to take time to talk with undivided attention. Maintaining intimacy requires investing in uninterrupted time together. Talking about day to day concerns is great, but happy couples also voice their fears and sadness, as well as hopes, dreams, and what brings them joy.

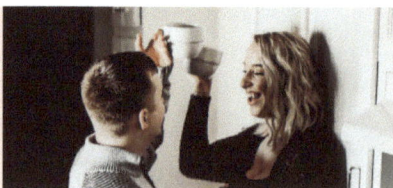

**LOVE HABIT # 15**

## CHEER

### When the world seems against you....

Happy couples know their partner has their back and is cheering them on to make their dreams a reality.

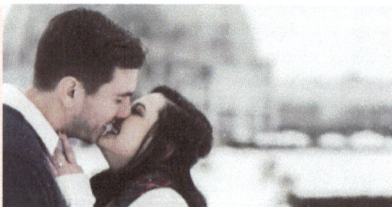

**LOVE HABIT # 16**

## CHERISH

### Even after all these years together...

Happy couples cherish each other and the time they get to spend together. They don't treat each other like an emotional garbage can at the end of a long and stressful day. Instead, they ask and give time and space to wind down in other ways.

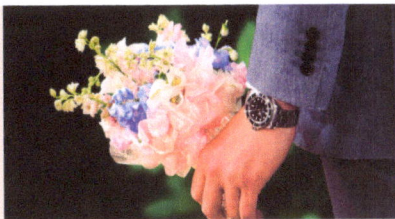

LOVE HABIT # 17
## SMALL SIGNS

### What is your partner's love language?
What makes your partner feel your love the most? Is it through acts of service, physical touch, gifts, quality time together, or words of affirmation? According to Gary Chapman, happy relationships don't require extravagant gifts. Instead, happy couples need to know the love language of their partner and focus on making small signs of their love in this language daily.

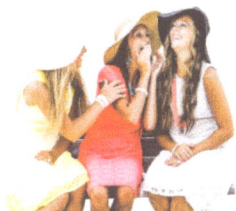

LOVE HABIT # 18
## SUPPORT NETWORK

### Do you have the support...
Of family, friends, and your community? A secret of happy couples is that they have a wider network that supports them when life gets tough. All of the love doesn't just fall on each other's shoulders. Instead, happy couples can also turn to friends, family, and neighbors for connection, support, and caring.

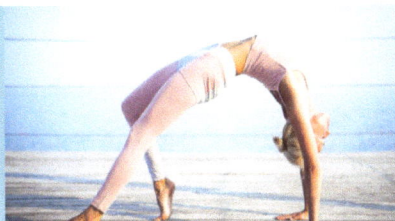

LOVE HABIT # 19
## SELF-LOVE

### The bliss starts with you....
Happy couples intuitively know that they are responsible for cultivating their own joy. They don't push responsibility for their happiness onto their partner. Instead, they invest in self-care and self-love which they then share with each other.

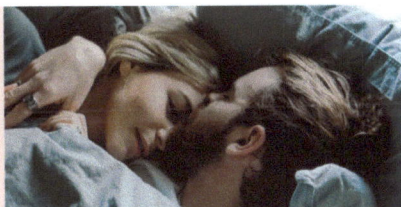

LOVE HABIT # 20
## FEEL UNIQUE

### Why play by the rules?
A secret of happy couples is they make their OWN love rules and habits to create trust, respect, intimacy, fun and blissful love. They don't try to imitate or compare themselves to other couples. Instead, they cherish the unique bond they are building and are devoted to working through tough times together.

*"It is not how much we do, but how much love we put in the doing. It is not how much we give, but how much love we put in the giving. Do ordinary things with extraordinary love." - Mother Teresa*

# Yoga for Friends or Lovers

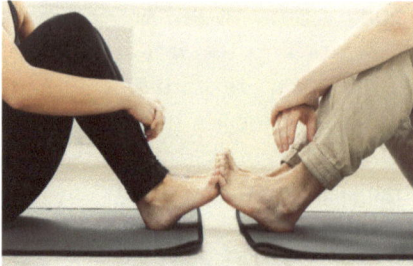

## Feet Kiss

-Bring the toes of the
feet to touch.
-Lengthen tailbone down and
engage low abs for a long spine.
-Look into each oth-
er's eyes while breathing
deeply for 2 minutes.

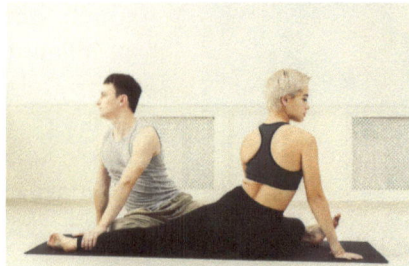

## Love Twist

-Face one another and both
bend the right knee in while
straightening the back leg.
-Inhale lengthen, twist
to the right and grab
your partner's ankle.
-Hold for 2 minutes
then switch sides.

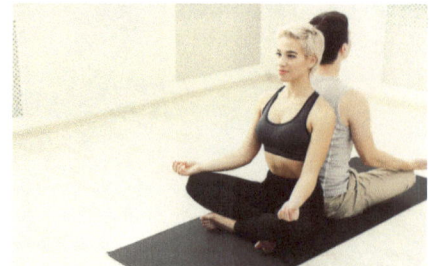

## Feel the Breath

-Bring your backs to-
gether to touch.
-Inhale lengthen the spine,
relax the shoulders, close the
eyes and breathe deeply.
-Feel the breath of your partner.
-Stay for 2-5 minutes.

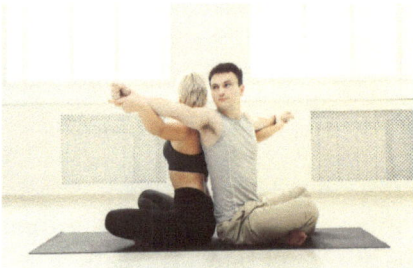

## Open the Heart

-Bring your backs to-
gether to touch.
-Inhale stretch your arms out
to shoulder height and clasp
your partner's hands gently.
-Twist slightly to the right
for 1 minute, then twist to
the left for 1 minute.

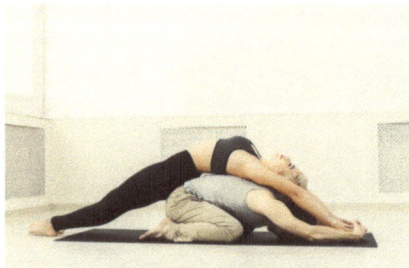

## Relax into Trust

-Sit back to back. 1 person folds
forward into Balasana, forehead on the floor or a block.
-Person 2 sits at their partner's
heels and gently leans back,
clasping hands and open-
ing the heart for 2 minutes.

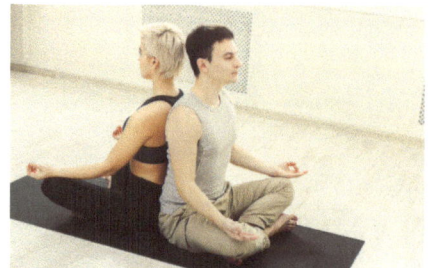

## Loving Kindness

-Bring your backs to-
gether to touch.
-Inhale lengthen the spine, relax
the shoulders, breathe deeply.
-Send warm, loving energy
from your heart into the body
of your partner for 2 minutes.

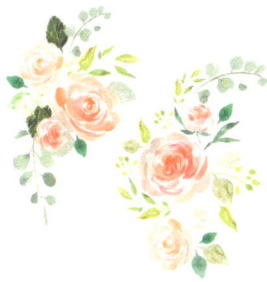

# What are the
# HABITS OF FRIENDSHIPS THAT LAST?

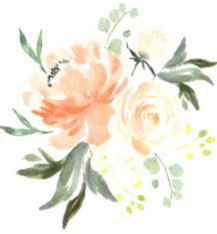

Do you want to build friendships that last the test of time? You're not alone. Most people are looking for a sense of belonging and connection. Research by Harvard following men over decades revealed that their most significant source of happiness came not from fame or fortune, but from their relationships. What is the easiest way to start building close friendships that last? Start being a good friend. Practice the habits of those who have maintained friendships over the decade.

**LOVE HABIT # 1**

## Generosity of Heart

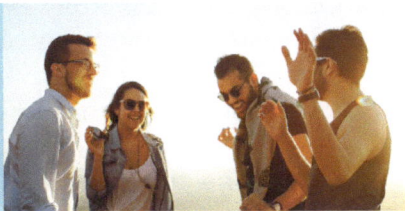

Strong friendships that last a lifetime connect two hearts. You celebrate each other's victories and support each other in times of frustration and failure.

**LOVE HABIT # 2**

## Patience Over Perfect

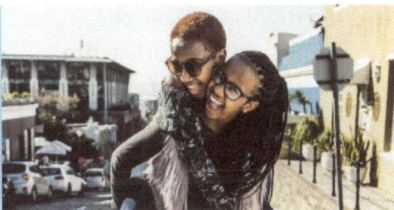

Arguments, misunderstandings, and mistakes can pull two friends apart. You don't need to kick a friendship to the curb when things get tough. Sometimes, friends need to seek out reconciliation. Other times it is wise to give the relationship a bit of 'breathing room' before coming back together again.

**LOVE HABIT # 3**

## APOLOGIZE & FORGIVE

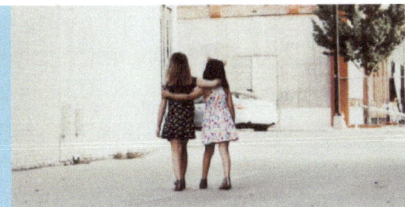

Can you ask for and GIVE forgiveness? One secret of friendships that last is that they make a habit of acknowledging they made a mistake and asking for forgiveness. They take action to make reparations. On the flip side, good friends can forgive one another faster and easier because they trust an apology is heartfelt.

**LOVE HABIT # 4**

**POSITIVITY**

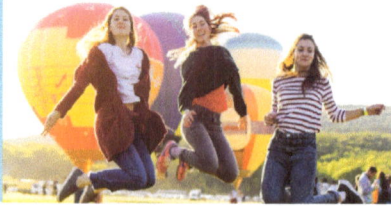

Strong friendships make it a habit to focus on the positive. They steer away from the jagged rocks of gossip. Negativity and complaining have little airing space. Instead of circling over problems and recriminations, the focus is on helping one another to release negative emotions, seize back personal power and search for solutions.

**LOVE HABIT # 5**

**EMPATHETIC LISTENING**

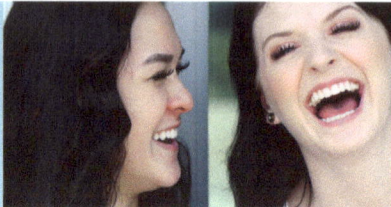

Friendships that last understand how critical it is to listen with their full attention and heart. They make a habit of putting away their digital devices and showing up with total concentration for their friends. Instead of crafting a response, or filtering what they are hearing through their narrative, outstanding friends quiet their thoughts.

**LOVE HABIT #**
**6**

**NO NARCISSIM**

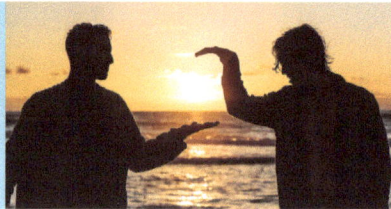

Friendships that last a lifetime reject narcissism. One person, no matter how charming or talented, cannot be the focus of the relationship for a bond to endure. Each has equal stage time to talk while the other listens attentively. Each friend is happy to take a step back and let the other shine in their moment of triumph.

**LOVE HABIT # 7**

**TRUST**

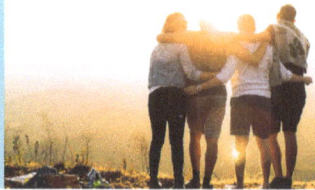

Friendships strong enough to last are built on trust. When hardship hits, the friend is there, no questions asked, to lend a hand or open their arms. Over a lifetime the repeated showing up to help when the going gets tough builds love and appreciation that can withstand storms of misunderstanding and arguments.

**LOVE HABIT # 8**

**COMPLIMENT**

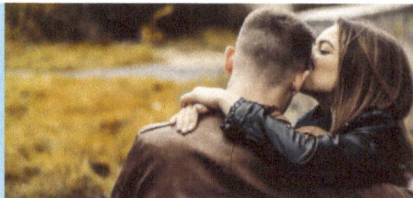

You need to be able to compliment and say no to build a strong friendship that lasts. Setting clear boundaries and communicating how you are prioritizing your life is kind. People and life situations change and friends that last support each other to evolve, grow, and learn. They compliment progress and support change.

## LOVE HABIT # 9
### USE HUMOR

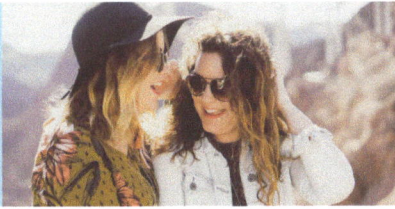

Laughter releases endorphins in the brain. Friends that laugh together can associate each other with regular doses of feel-good chemicals. A secret habit of happy friendships is their use of humor in a fight. Friends use humor to defuse a fight when negative emotions get too much.

## LOVE HABIT # 10
### CREATE ANNUAL RITUALS

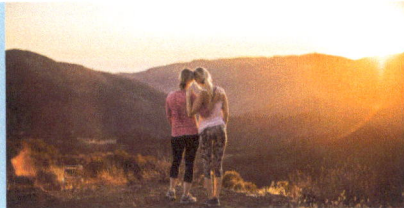

A habit of friendships that last a lifetime is regular meetings. It could be enjoying a coffee every week, or meeting for lunch once a month. It could be traveling to celebrate the 4th of July together every year, or going on the annual yoga retreat the first weekend of June.

## LOVE HABIT # 11
### AUTHENTIC

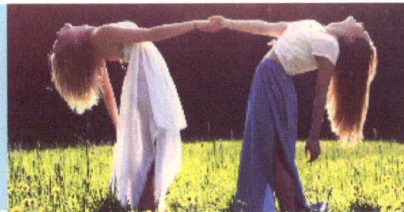

Sure, you may want to paint a perfect picture on social media. With friends, you need to be honest. It doesn't mean you need to dwell on the trauma or unpleasant issues. Admitting to weaknesses, sadness, fears, or hardships will make you more human. The intimacy of opening up will make the good times sweeter.

## LOVE HABIT # 12
### REJECT JEALOUSY

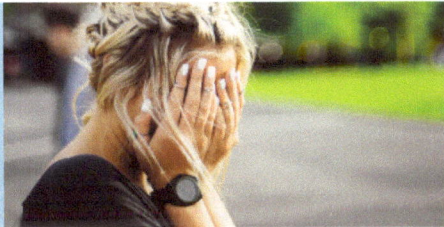

Jealousy has no space in a friendship that lasts a lifetime. Real friends don't feel the need to downplay their accomplishments, talents, strengths, or good fortune. They know their good friend wants the best for them in life. If jealousy does rear its ugly face, you show it to the door.

## LOVE HABIT # 13
### SHOW ME THE LOVE

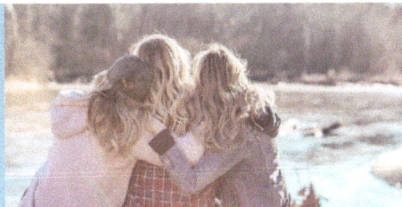

To build a friendship that lasts there needs to be an appreciation for each other. Compliments are the perfect preventative medicine in some relationships. In other bonds, the secret sauce is affection, gratitude, gifts, or little acts of service.

# Emotional & Spiritual Wellness Evaluation / Affirmations

| | Highly disagree | Disagree | Slightly disagree | Slightly agree | Agree | Strongly agree |
|---|---|---|---|---|---|---|
| • Usually I feel in control of my emotions. | | | | | | |
| • Usually I am joyful and happy. | | | | | | |
| • I am rarely depressed or low. | | | | | | |
| • I have a high level of integrity between what I think, say, and do. | | | | | | |
| • My attitude towards life is consistently positive. | | | | | | |
| • I feel very much in control of my own life. | | | | | | |
| • Stress or anxiety plague me seldom. | | | | | | |
| • I can elucidate clearly the emotions that are most valuable to me. | | | | | | |
| • I have spent time reflecting on how I want to feel and show up in the world. | | | | | | |
| • I have spent time reflecting and know my values and can tell them to you. | | | | | | |
| • I know I can handle the challenges of life and retain an inner strength. | | | | | | |
| • I believe I deserve to be content and experience joy. | | | | | | |
| • I know what a person of integrity is, says, and does. | | | | | | |
| • I act to make things happen in my life versus letting things happen. | | | | | | |
| • I can treat what arises with equanimity - with calm. | | | | | | |
| • I pause between triggers and my response to them. | | | | | | |

| | Highly disagree | Disagree | Slightly disagree | Slightly agree | Agree | Strongly agree |
|---|---|---|---|---|---|---|
| • I am very content most of the time. | | | | | | |
| • I believe in a power I can turn to greater than me. | | | | | | |
| • I have a sense of my purpose in life; I can articulate it. | | | | | | |
| • I can articulate my spiritual beliefs. | | | | | | |
| • I feel very fulfilled as a human being. | | | | | | |
| • I live consciously and pay attention to all areas of my life. | | | | | | |
| • I seek out inspirational or uplifting books, media | | | | | | |
| • I make the world a better place and contribute. | | | | | | |
| • I am accepting of all parts of myself, both good and bad. | | | | | | |
| • I am pursuing new ideas to live my best life. | | | | | | |
| • I have thought deeply about my quality of life and defined exactly what a beautiful life means for me versus culture, marketing, family, or friends' definitions. | | | | | | |
| • I deserve the best life has to offer. | | | | | | |
| • I travel often and can go with the flow, enjoying the unexpected. I am open to surprise. | | | | | | |
| • I have a lot of fun in my life. | | | | | | |
| • I feel that I am truly living my life to the fullest. | | | | | | |
| • I plan extraordinary experiences on an ongoing basis, creating memorable moments. | | | | | | |
| • The majority of the objects in my life spark joy. | | | | | | |
| • I have a vision for how I would like my life to unfold over the coming years. | | | | | | |
| • I am acting on a plan to improve an area of my wellness and achieve my ideal life. | | | | | | |
| • I am dedicated to improving my life in every area. | | | | | | |
| • I want to continue to grow and develop. | | | | | | |

# Greet the day. Rising

Getting better sleep and starting your day with energy begins with regulating your rising time. Aim to get up at around the same time each morning and going to bed at the same time at night.

Do you leap out of bed in the morning full of energy? Or is it an effort to stumble out of bed and toward the kitchen for a jolt of caffeine?

Either way, you can turn your morning into a source of profound well-being. Starting your day with space for hydration, movement, focus, inspiration, and silence will transform every aspect of your life. Set aside a minimum of twenty-five minutes in the morning to devote to your new morning revitalize routine.

*"Health is the greatest possession. Contentment is the greatest treasure. Confidence is the greatest friend. Non-being is the greatest joy." - Lao Tzu*

## MORNING REVITALIZE FOR BEGINNERS

Do you have a habit of reaching for a cup of coffee first thing in the morning? Wait until after your morning revitalize routine, or at least until step four. That aromatic cup of bliss may be what keeps you from starting or finishing your revitalize routine. Use your favorite cup of coffee or tea as your celebration after completing your new method for greeting the day.

Would you like to boost your energy, vitality, mind-focus, and natural glow?

### Glow Water Therapy

1. Go to the kitchen and squeeze half of a fresh lemon into half a liter of water and drink.
2. Drink your second glass of water forty-five minutes after your first glass.

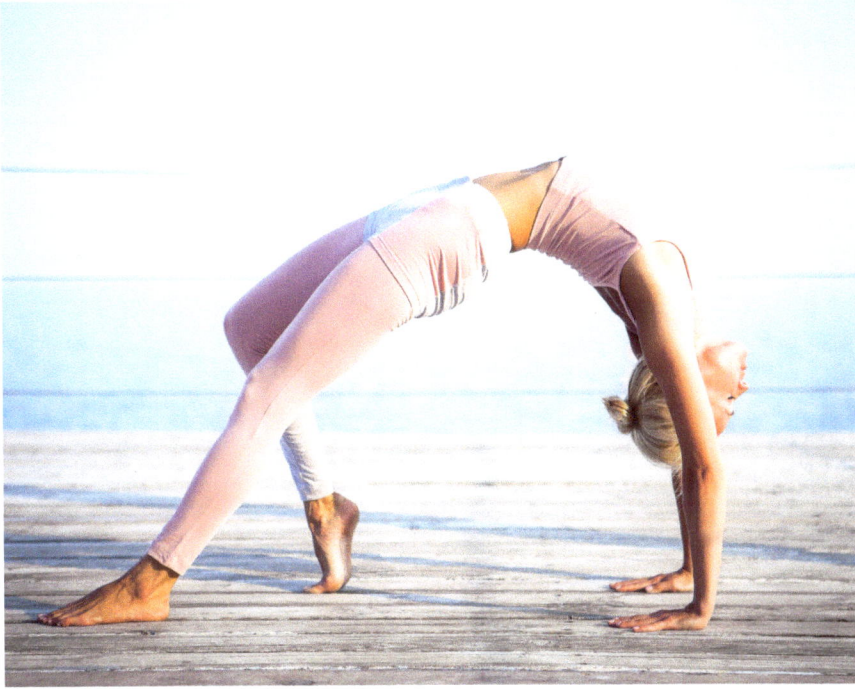

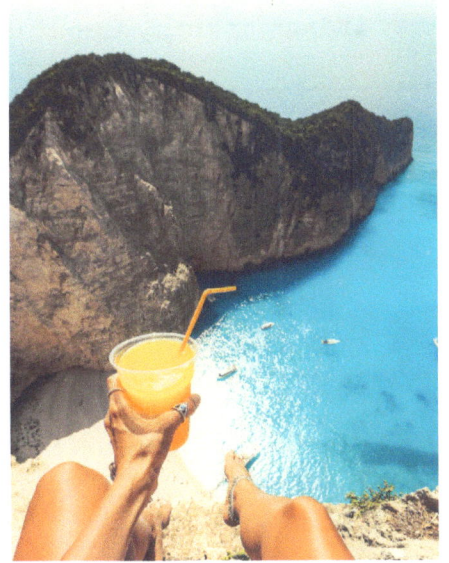

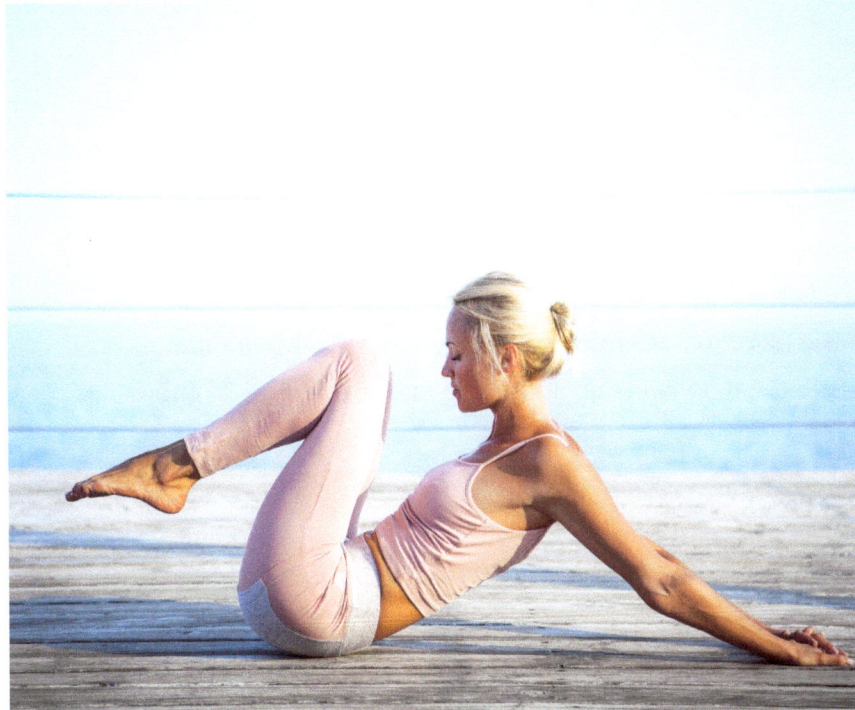

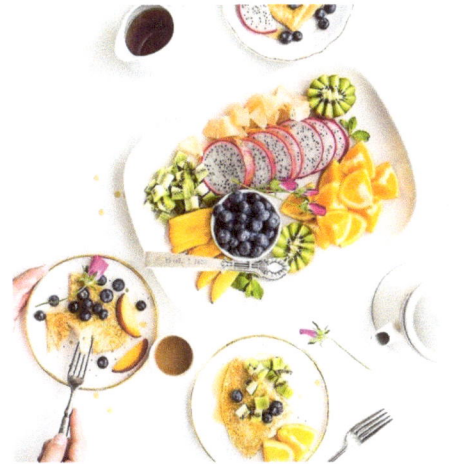

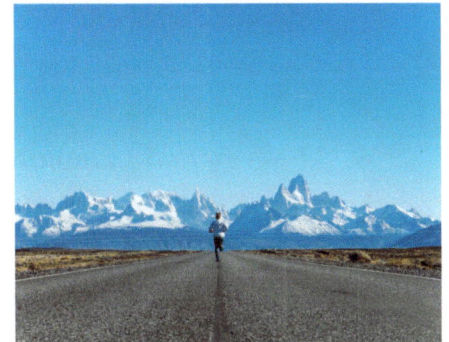

## Water Therapy Benefits:

### 1.  Flush toxins from the body.

Your body produces waste as it repairs and cleans itself during slumber. When you awake, you are dehydrated. Drinking a liter of water on an empty stomach enables this waste to flow out of the body through your urine. The antioxidant properties found in the lemon juice aide in the elimination of toxins from the blood and body.

### 2.  Balances your pH and increases well-being.

The lemon juice in your early morning water therapy becomes alkaline in your stomach and works to balance your pH levels. Properly balanced pH improves your skin glow, digestion, absorption of nutrients, and release of toxins from your body.

### 3.  Primes your body to absorb nutrients easier.

A purified and hydrated digestion system and colon will enable you to absorb nutrients better.

### 4.  Weight loss and healthy weight maintenance.

Water therapy revs up your metabolism by up to 25% in the morning, reduces constipation, and improves your digestion. You will feel less bloated and lighter.

### 5.  Skin glowing with natural health.

Hydration aids the body in purging itself of toxins. Instead of being pulled to the digestion tract and organs, hydration can flow to the skin and give you a healthy glow. The fresh lemon you squeeze in your water fights radicals that cause wrinkles and aging and is effective at improving the look and even texture of your skin.

### 6.  Energy and Immunity Boost.

Following the Glow Water Therapy daily for a few weeks will sky-rocket your energy levels and boost your immunity as the early morning hyper-hydration balances your lymph system.

### 7.  Improved focus and concentration.

Dehydration causes headaches and a lack of an ability to focus. By starting your day at maximum hydration, you are consuming the fluid you need for your brain to concentrate better.

## 8.   Will wake you up better than coffee.

As unbelievable as it may sound, the Glow Water Therapy wakes you up better than a cup of coffee can. The hydration enables your body to send water to the brain, flush out toxins, and prime and purify the digestion system. You will experience an increase in alertness like drinking a cup of coffee, but you will also experience a higher sense of vitality and well-being you don't get from your favorite coffee drink.

   NOTE: Too much of a good thing can hurt you. Drinking too much water can even kill you. How much is too much? Never drink more than a liter in an hour. Incorporate this simple Glow Water Therapy into your daily routine to power-up your health and wellness and increase your concentration for higher productivity at work.

# MORNING REVITALIZE STEPS

## STEP 1: HYDRATE (2 MINUTES)

Jump out of bed the moment your alarm goes off in the morning. Slice a lemon in half and squeeze it into half a liter of water. Drink down the entire glass. Refill and carry it with you.

## STEP 2: MOVEMENT (10 MINUTES)

Yoga, tai chi, or qi gong first thing in the morning will allow the energy in your body to flow, your metabolism to rev up, and your mind and body to become alert and ready for the day. The linking of deep, slow breathing with movement can pull you into the present moment.  Not only will you be increasing your flexibility, strength, and physical health, but these types of exercise prepare you for your day in subtle ways.

   A calm, quiet mind is less reactive, more resilient to stress, and primed for creativity and concentration. Do you think it is impossible to roll out of bed and onto a yoga mat without a cup of coffee? I felt that way too. I promise energy movement flows like yoga will awaken your body and mind better than a cup of coffee. Do you think you need to get sweaty in a high cardio workout for at least 20 minutes to improve your health, well-being, and physical fitness? I thought that too. It turns out that just ten minutes of yoga in the morning can lead to weight loss, an improvement in health, and a spike in well-being.

Deep, slow, rhythmic breathing is the essential ingredient in yoga, tai chi, and qi gong. Otherwise, you are just doing gymnastics or aerobics. The breath is where the magic happens. Most people breathe short, shallow breaths. When stressed, this breathing becomes even more rapid. Deep, slow breathing turns the stress response in the body off and the parasympathetic nervous system on. The parasympathetic nervous system is the repair and care mode in the body. Circulation increases, digestion flows, cell repair, and an immune system boost occur when the parasympathetic nervous system is turned on. Close your mouth and begin to breathe in and out your nose. Place your hands on your belly.

### INHALATION.

Breathe into your stomach, causing your hands to rise. Exhale and feel your hands lower. Try this for five breaths. Next, place one hand on your belly and one hand over your heart. Breathe into your stomach and then expand your lungs in 360 degrees, causing your heart to lift beneath your hand. The hand over your belly will rise and then the hand over your heart lift on your deep, slow inhalation.

### EXHALATION.

Keep one hand on your belly and one hand over your heart. Aim now to breathe out the nose as slowly and smoothly as you can. The hand over the heart should lower first, then the hand over your belly.

Towards the end of your exhalation pull the belly actively in the direction of your spine and up under your ribcage as you lift the pelvic floor. Lifting the pelvic floor means squeezing the same muscles you use to stop the flow of urine. Engaging the muscles to pull the belly in expels all air from the lungs and strengthens your core. Focus on this exhalation for five breaths. Now you're ready to add on constricting the back of your throat on each exhalation. Slightly tightening the muscles of the throat as you exhale produces a wave-like sound in the throat.

### THE RESULT.

Now put it all together. Inhale slowly and deeply through the nose. Feel your belly rise, then your

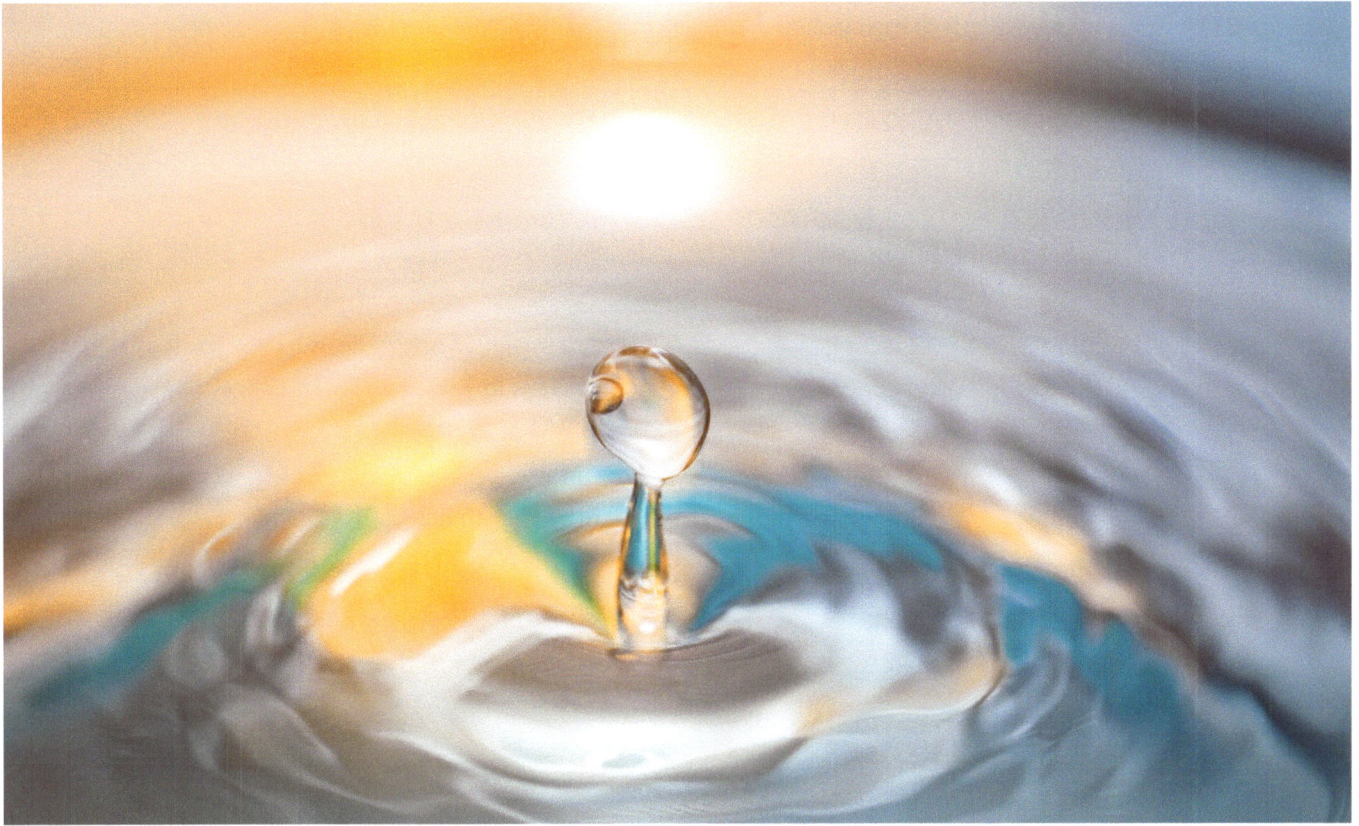

"You are not a drop in the ocean.
You are the entire ocean, in a drop." – Rumi

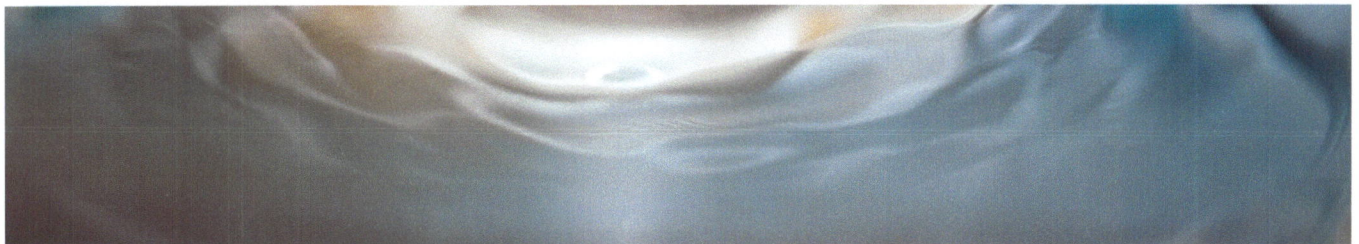

chest lift. Exhale slowly out the nose. Feel your chest lower, your belly relaxes as you engage the pelvic floor and actively pull the belly button in towards the spine and up under the ribcage. Use this breathing method throughout your yoga, tai chi, or qi gong practice. At the end of your flow of movement drink your second glass of water.

## STEP 3: FOCUS (3 MINUTES)

Find a quiet space where you will not be disturbed. Have a pillow or cushion ready for five minutes of focus. Sit down on the floor with crossed legs and bring the cushion under your sitting bones, so your hips are higher than your knees.

In this comfortable seat, lengthen the spine and soften the front ribs inwards as you melt the shoulder blades down your back. Sit up even taller, lengthening the spine, lifting the top of your head higher. You will find sitting with a long spine challenging. Another option is to bring your back to a wall so you can sit with a tall spine, or sit in a straight-backed chair instead. Set a timer of five minutes. Begin to cultivate a deep, slow, even breath through the nose.

## MEDITATION 1: FEEL INTO THE BODY

Place your right hand in your lap. Rest the left hand on top of the right. Bring your thumbs to touch. Close your eyes. On your inhalation visualize a golden light traveling up your feet, throughout your entire body and out the crown of your head. On the expiration see the light, like sunshine, moving down through the top of your head and flowing down through every corner of your body before exiting the soles of your feet.

Thoughts will drag your attention away. When you realize this has happened, don't get frustrated. Don't judge. Just return your attention once again to the breath and the traveling of the golden light up and down through your body.

## MEDITATION 2: LOVE EQUANIMITY

Bring your right hand to rest over your heart. Rest the left hand on top of the right. Begin to pray or send energy and love out to people in your life. Start first with those you love most dearly. Bring the first person to mind. Mentally say, "I wish you health, happiness, and peace."

"If you realize that all things change, there is nothing you will try to hold on to. If you are not afraid of dying, there is nothing you cannot achieve." -Lao Tzu

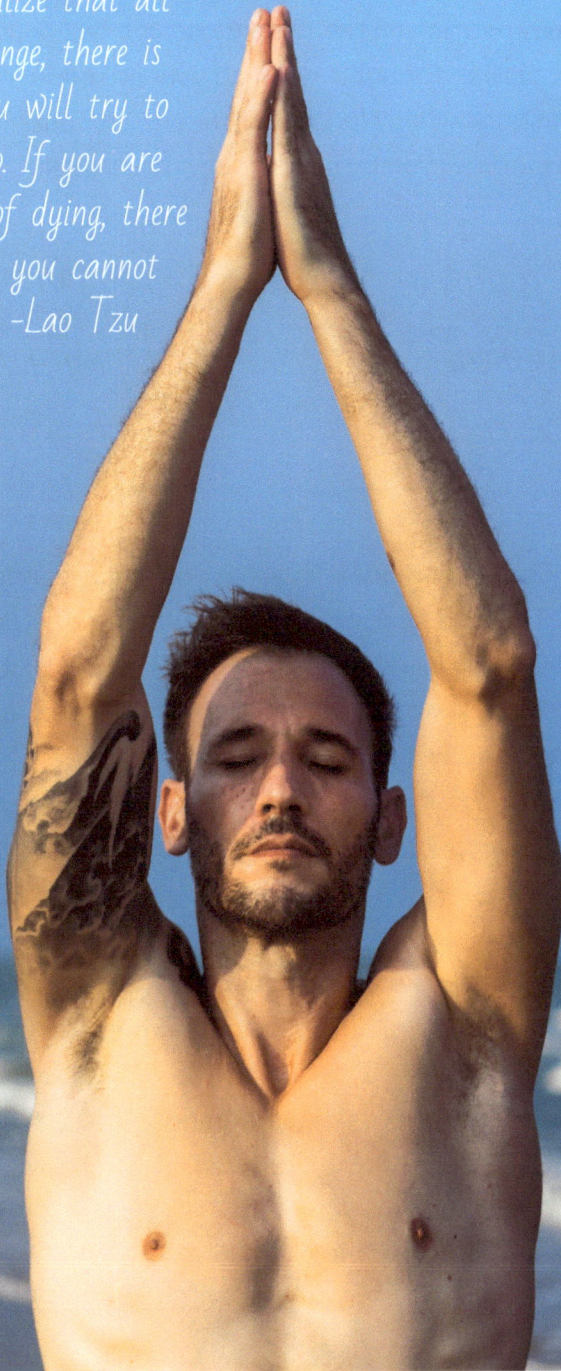

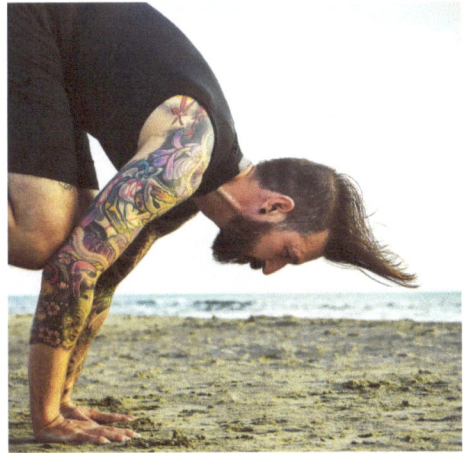

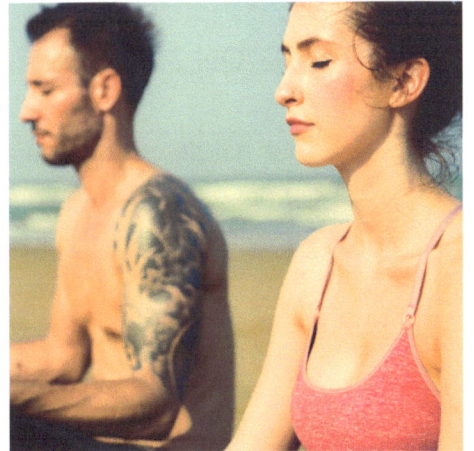

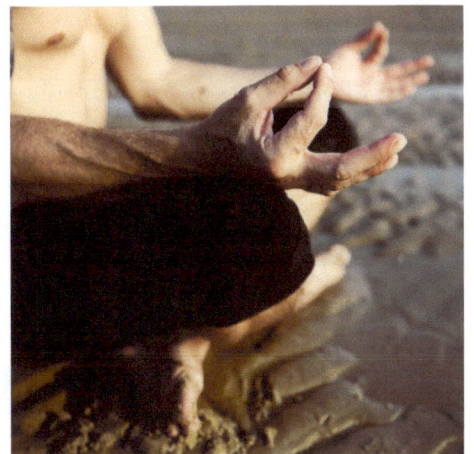

Alternatively, you can say, "I pray you are healthy, happy, at peace." As you internally say these words, try to feel the love flowing out from your heart towards this person. Repeat with each person you love deeply. Next, proceed with people you like, then those you feel neutral. Finish with people you find challenging or actively dislike. Thoughts will drag your attention away. When you realize this has happened, don't get frustrated. Don't judge. Just return your attention once again to the breath and on sending love outwards. Finish by sending love to yourself.

*"The chariot of the mind is drawn by wild horses, and those wild horses have to be tamed." –Svetasvatara Upanishad*

## MEDITATION 3: MANTRA

Rest your hands out on your knees. Touch your index finger to your thumb. Alternatively, rest your hands, palms up, on your thighs. On each inhalation, focus on the word HUM. Every exhalation repeat the word SA internally. You do not need to speak the words aloud. HUM and SA are in Sanskrit. The benefit of focusing on Sanskrit words is it is unlikely you have emotions attached to them. Feel free to select your own two words if this will serve you better.

You could focus on the word PEACE on the in breath and JOY on the out breath. Thoughts, sounds, or bodily distractions will drag your attention away. When you realize this has happened, don't get frustrated. Don't judge. Just return your attention once again to your mantra and the breath. When five minutes is done, open your eyes, bow forward to rebound your energy, smile, and then stand up slowly, so as not to disturb the tranquility you have activated in your mind and body.

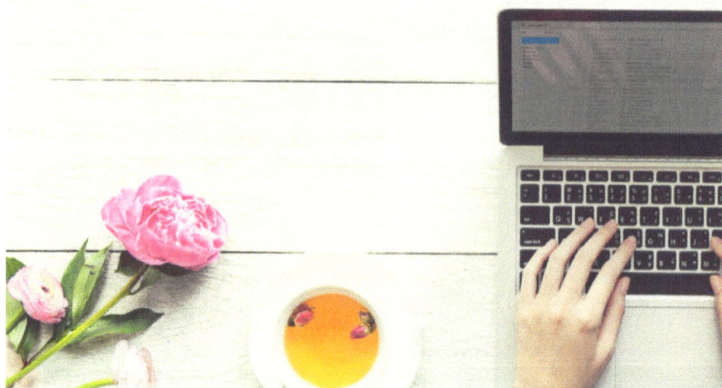

## STEP 4: INSPIRATION & LEARNING (10 MINUTES)

In the busy, hectic, or repetitive mundane of life, we can lose touch with our inner craving for creativity and learning. You can infuse your life with inspiration. Just set aside as little as ten minutes in the morning to create or learn something you find interesting and that sparks joy. The key is to release attachment to the end result while giving your full effort each day during these five minutes. Most of us live in a culture attached to goals and achievements. Working with passion and surrendering clinging or hoping to an end outcome may feel challenging and bizarre.

Just remind yourself that the intention is to cultivate more inspiration in your life by stoking the fires of creativity, curiosity, and passion.

So what can you do with just ten minutes? First, decide on your project. What would you like to learn or create? A multitude of free and inexpensive courses are available today. Try not to select a class that is practical, but preferably one that ignites excitement. Perhaps you have always wanted to learn Italian, meditation, positive psychology, coding, or the history of ancient civilizations. If you have decided that you are not artistic in the past, release this pressure.

You may find coloring in an adult coloring book or paint by numbers profoundly satisfying. You don't have to create artwork to sell or showcase. Getting into and enjoying the creative flow is the intention, whether it is through painting, drawing, coloring, sculpting, designing, writing, sewing, knitting, crafting, cooking, or baking.

No one needs to see the result but you. During these ten minutes work in as much silence as you can — turn off music, television, and background noise. Silence can be uncomfortable at first if you are accustomed to constant noise. Lean into the discomfort. Reacquaint yourself with silence, which can have a healing effect on the mind and body.

Ten minutes a day may not sound like enough time. Believe me when I say that those few minutes will add up. By the end of the week, you will have invested seventy minutes into learning or creating. You will set a different tone for your entire day by beginning with a dose of inspiration.

## STEP 1: HYDRATE (2 MINUTES)

## STEP 2: MOVEMENT (10 MINUTES)

## STEP 3: FOCUS (3 MINUTES)

## STEP 4: INSPIRATION & LEARNING (10 MINUTES)

## HABIT STACKING

Smooth flowing from hydration to movement, focus, and inspiration in silence will take practice. The key is always to follow the same routine. Going from drinking your lemon water straight to flowing with movement, then sitting for meditation or prayer, and following with learning or creating will become easy.

Stacking these habits in this specific order means you will need to summon far less will-power. Instead of invoking change in one area of your life, you will be doing so in four ways at one go. To begin, try not to miss a single day of your revitalize morning routine for twenty-one days in a row. You will be creating the mental groove to set new wellness morning on auto-pilot. What happens if life gets in the way and you miss out on your revitalize morning routine? Relax. Flow through each element throughout your day with what is available.

Do you have a five am flight? Drink your half a liter of water as soon as you get to the airport, for instance, then activate your yoga breathing while you walk through the airport terminal for ten minutes, focusing on your breath.

Find a quiet space to meditate or pray for a few minutes, and close by engaging in ten minutes of learning or creativity on the plane. You may not have access to your current project, but brainstorm something new you can learn or create at the airport. With just a pen and paper you could write a letter, sketch a drawing, or create an original recipe.

*"We are what we repeatedly do. Excellence, then, is not an act, but a habit." -Aristotle*

## MORNING REVITALIZE FOR PARENTS

You may not be able to wake up before your baby or children. You're just too tired, or no matter how early you set your alarm clock, they seem to get up also. Don't despair. You can complete your morning revitalize routine during your babies morning nap. If you have small children, you can flow through your routine (most likely with some interruptions), after you have attended to their needs, first. You can then inform your children as to your new morning routine and ask that they give you this time.

You may think it impossible that a two-year-old will understand or respect your request.

Don't be surprised if they calmly play with their toys next to you, join in trying to do the yoga, or curl up in your lap silently during prayer or meditation. You can incorporate your child into your inspiration step. Your child may even learn Italian faster than you do or beg you to extend the painting time. Your children will begin to notice the change in you from engaging in these twenty-five minutes of wellness before you even do. They will want the more vibrant parent they get afterward and begin to love the routine as much as you do.

*"I know of no more encouraging fact than the unquestionable ability of man to elevate his life by conscious endeavor." —Henry David Thoreau*

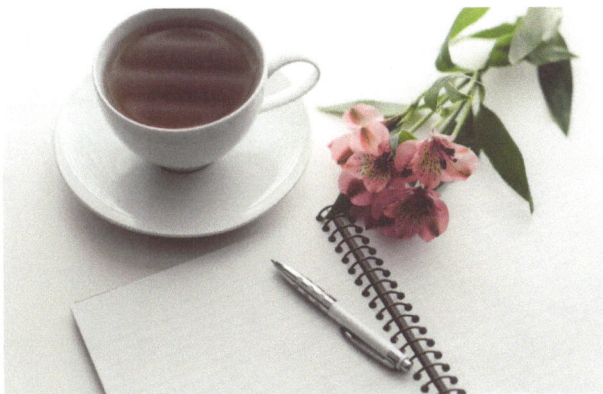

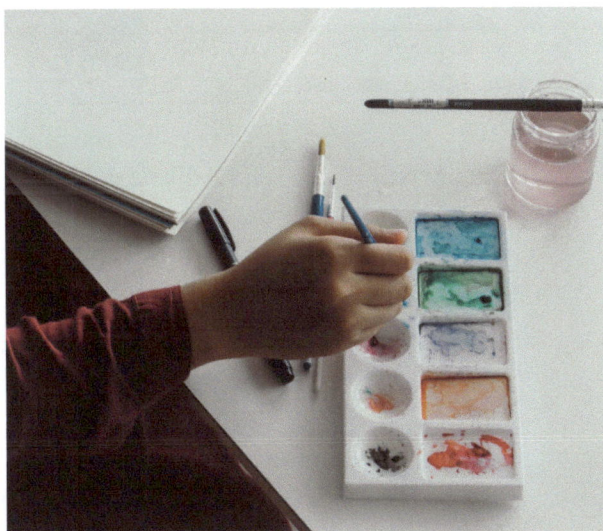

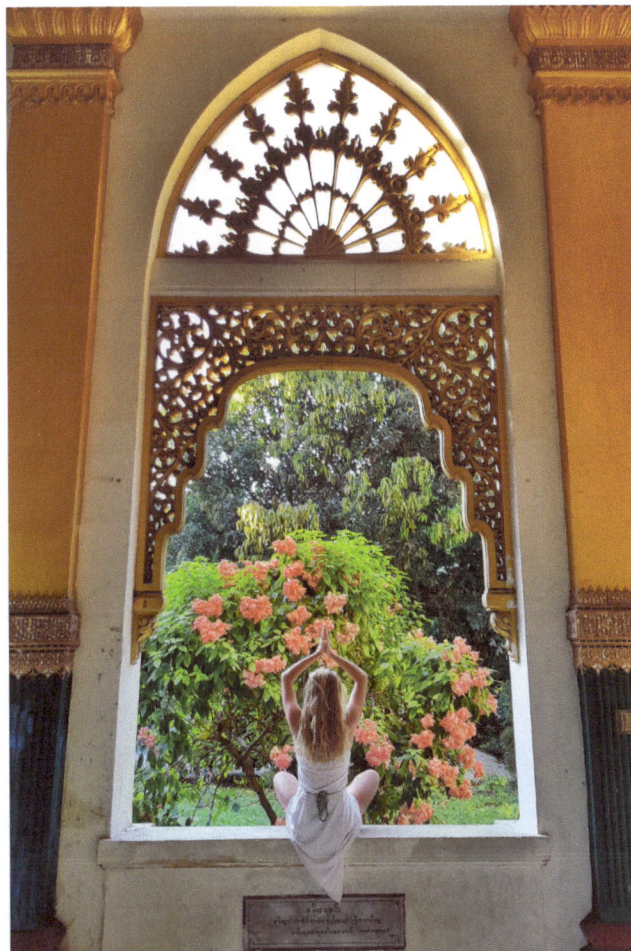

# Yoga Flow to WAKE UP & ENERGIZE

**1**

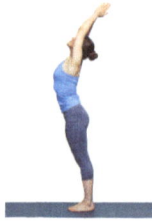

## Tadasana

-Press into all four corners of the feet.
-Shoulders over hips.
-Lengthen tailbone down and engage low abs for a long spine.
-Hands sweep up.

**2**

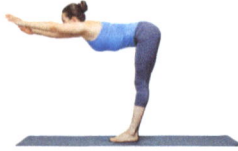

## Ardha Uttanasana

-Spread the arms out as you fold over your legs. Head drops last.
-Inhale, lengthen, look forward, pull abs in.
-Lift pelvic floor.
-Fold over your legs.

**3**

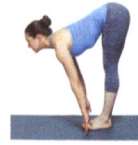

## Uttanasana

-Spread the arms out as you fold over your legs. Head drops last.
-Inhale lengthen, look forward, pull abs in.
-Lift pelvic floor.
-Fold over your legs.

**4**

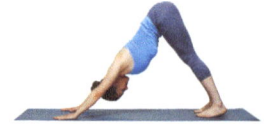

## Adho Mukha

-Spread fingers wide.
-Press the hips back as push out of the arms.
-Lengthen the spine.
-Melt the heels down.
-Lift pelvic floor.
-Pull the belly inwards.

**5**

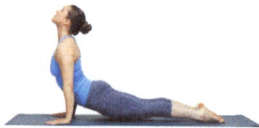

## Urdhva Mukha

-Lift the heart forward and through the arms.
-Press into the tops of the feet. Lift the legs.
-Roll shoulders back and down the spine.
-Micro-bend the arms.

**6**

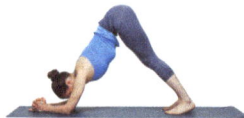

## Prep Pincha Mayurasana

-Ground forearms shoulder width apart.
-Curl toes under. Straighten the legs.
-Lift one leg up and then the other.

**7**

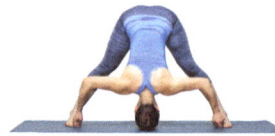

## Prasarita Padottanasana

-Grab your big toes.
-Fold forward in between your legs.
-Engage the legs.
-Lengthen the spine.
-Use the abs to fold.

**8**

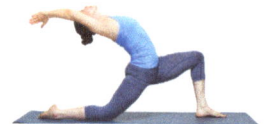

## Anjaneyasana

-Left knee over ankle.
-Lower right knee to the mat.
-Sweep the arms out and up, lifting up out of the low back.
-Soften the ribs.

Hold each pose for 3-5 deep, slow, even breaths with sound in and out the nose, creating a wave like sound with your breathing by constricting the back of the throat. Repeat the flow with the right leg and then relax in Shavasana for 5-10 minutes.

| 9 | 10 | 11 | 12 |
|---|---|---|---|

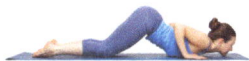 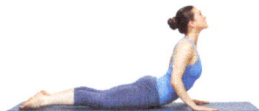 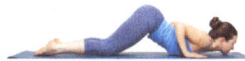 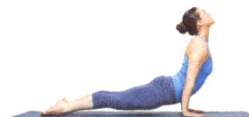

### Chaturanga

-Stack shoulders over wrists. Lower knees to the mat. Look forward.
-Squeeze elbows into the ribcage as you lower down.
-Keep shoulders back.

### Bhujangasana

-Place hands by chest.
-Lift the heart forward and through the arms.
-Press into the tops of the feet. Active legs.
-Roll shoulders back and down the spine.

### Chaturanga

-Stack shoulders over wrists. Lower knees to the mat. Look forward.
-Squeeze elbows into the ribcage as you lower down.
-Keep shoulders back.

### Urdhva Mukha

-Lift the heart forward and through the arms.
-Press into the tops of the feet. Lift the legs.
-Roll shoulders back and down the spine.
-Micro-bend the arms.

| 13 | 14 | 15 | 16 |
|---|---|---|---|

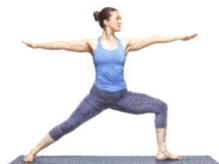 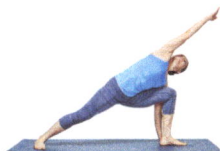 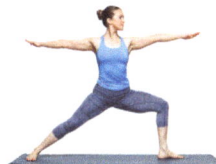 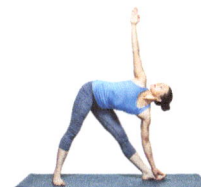

### Virabhadrasana II

-Ground the left foot between the hands.
-Pivot the right foot down and lift up.
-Stack shoulders over hips. Lift the heart.
-Pelvic floor lift.

### Parsvakonasana

-Left knee over left ankle. Draw the right arm over the right ear.
-Roll left hip under.
-Stretch from the edge of the right foot up through the fingers.

### Virabhadrasana II

-Lift back up to warrior II..
-Pivot the right foot down and lift up.
-Stack shoulders over hips. Lift the heart.
-Pelvic floor lift.

### Trikonasana

-Straighten the front leg with a micro-bend in the knee.
-Pull the front hip back and lengthen the side body.
-Revolve open.

**17**

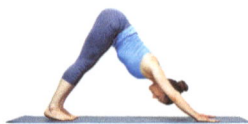

## Adho Mukha

-Spread fingers wide.
-Press the hips back as
push out of the arms.
-Lengthen the spine.
-Melt the heels down.
-Lift pelvic floor.
-Pull the belly inwards.

**18**

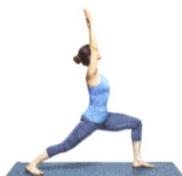

## Virabhadrasana I

-Right foot be-
tween the hands.
-Ground the edge of
the left foot down.
-Square the hips.
-Lift your arms up.
-Soften your ribs in.

**19**

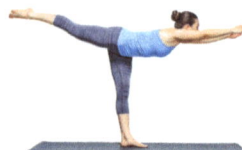

## Virabhadrasana III

-Ground into the left
foot as you lift the
right leg up behind
you, keeping hips
square to the front.
-Straight right leg.
-Reach arms forward.

**20**

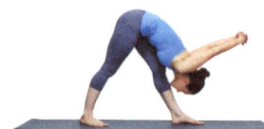

## Parsvottanasana

-Shorten your stance.
-Straighten both legs.
-Pull left hip back.
-Micro-bend left knee.
-Fold over your leg.
-Hands on floor or
blocks. Pull abs in.

**21**

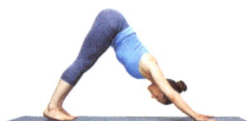

## Adho Mukha

-Spread fingers wide.
-Press the hips back as
push out of the arms.
-Lengthen the spine.
-Melt the heels down.
-Lift pelvic floor.
-Pull the belly inwards.

**22**

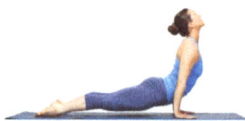

## Urdhva Mukha

-Lift the heart forward
and through the arms.
-Press into the tops of
the feet. Lift the legs.
-Roll shoulders back
and down the spine.
-Micro-bend the arms.

**23**

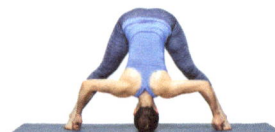

## Prasarita
## Padottanasana

-Grab your big toes.
-Fold forward in
between your legs.
-Engage the legs.
-Lengthen the spine.
-Use the abs to fold.

**24**

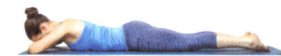

## Prone Shavasana

-Lower your fore-
head to rest on the
tops of your hands.
-Allow your entire
body to soften and
melt into the mat.
-Breathe with sound.

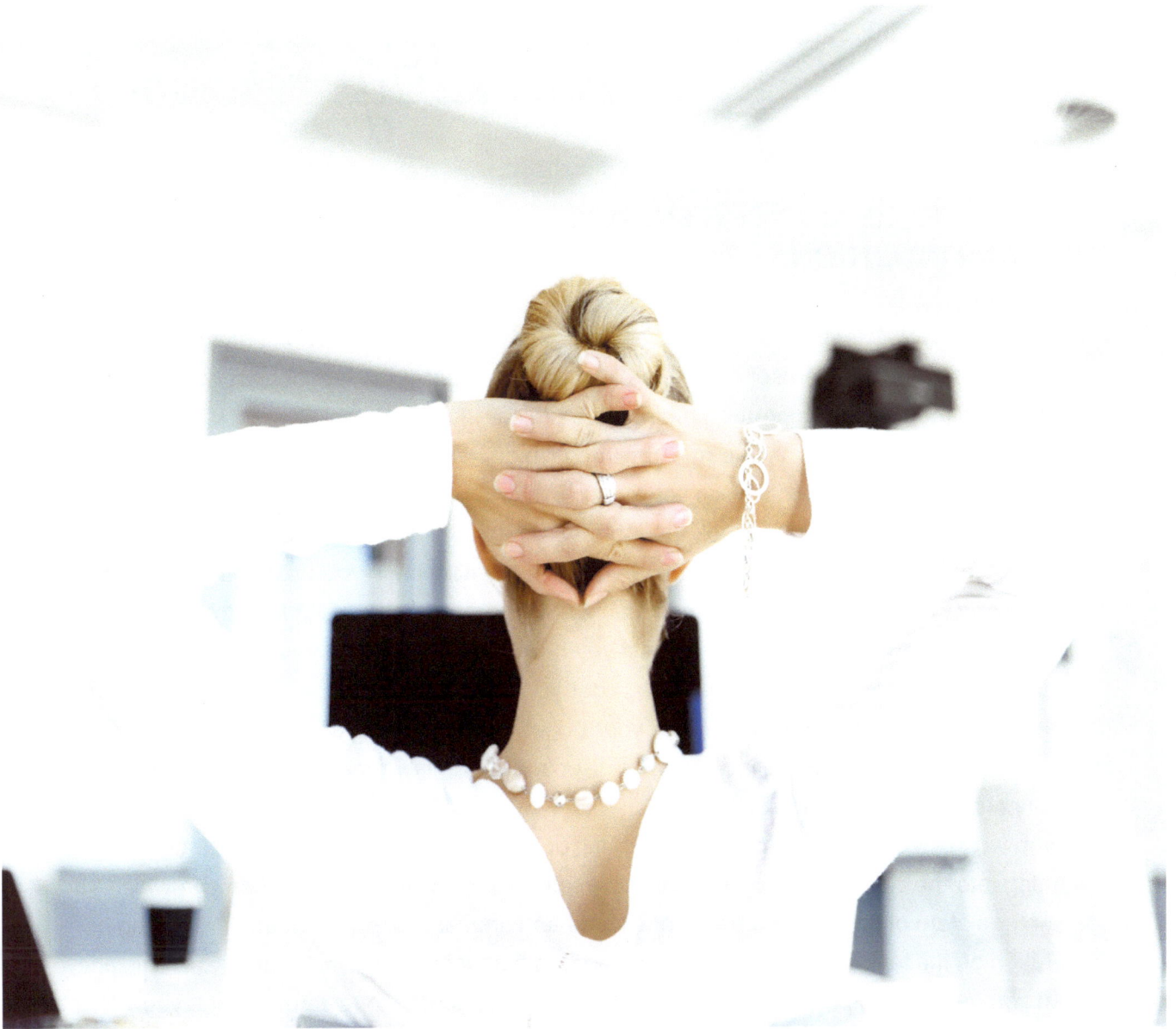

"Success is not the key to happiness.
Happiness is the key to success." - Albert Schweitzer, Noble Peace Prize Winner

# Wellness and joy while *Working*

## LEVERAGE EARLY MORNING ENERGY.
## SET YOUR INTENTION.

The embers of your creativity are still glowing from your revitalize morning sequence when you get to work. Leverage your inspiration, high energy, and focus in the first hour of work. Begin by working on a medium to a long-term project or a project that requires high creativity or focus.

On Sunday you planned out your medium, long-range, and top priority work, so you need not waste time with indecision or aimless activity.

Do not check your email and block the Internet if you can't resist checking social media, the news, or engaging in excessive research. Write down an intention for the next hour of work, such as, write one thousand words, write the meal plan and grocery list, create the strategy. Be specific. At the end of the hour stop. Sit down if you have been working on your feet.

Stand up if you have been sitting. Stretch out your legs as you check if you have met your target. Don't despair if you have not met your target. With time you will achieve your intention more often. If you have another hour at your disposal, set a new target for the second hour and set yourself to work again.

Some workplaces are so frantic, busy, and full of interruptions that you would be best served by going into the office early. You will earn yourself a full hour of undisturbed time in which you can enter a state of flow. Losing sense of all time and space, focusing with an unwavering concentration on the task in front of you, you will access higher creativity, inspiration, and efficiency. When you have accomplished work on a high priority, medium or long-term project, you will set a more vibrant and optimistic energy for the rest of your workday.

Attend in the second or third hour of your work day to your most arduous activity. What do you need to get done today to leave work in the evening satisfied? Get it done before lunchtime. Once again write down what you intend to accomplish during the hour. Set a timer and begin. When the timer chimes, review your progress and write it down. Be realistic and optimistic when writing down your intention for an hour of work. Most people have the attention of a goldfish.

Setting an intention for one hour of work, setting a timer, and blocking out as many distractions as possible will train your concentration muscles.

Few people understand the power of creating a clear intention and working towards it with laser-like focus. Within a few days, you will be surprised at how much more you are getting done with each hour. Don't be surprised if you start getting more done before lunch then you previously did in an entire workday.

*"He knew that Resistance was strongest at the finish. He did what he had to do, no matter how nutty or unorthodox, to finish and be ready to ship." - Steven Pressfield*

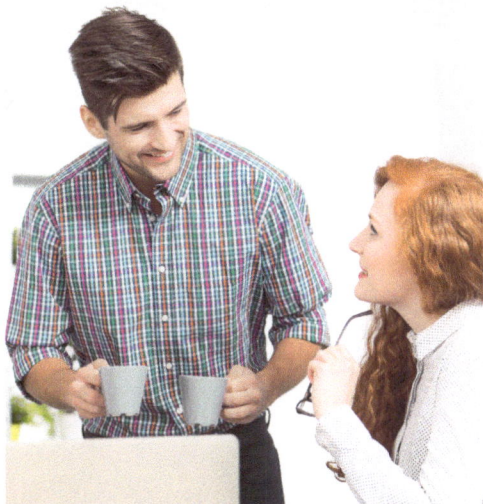

## KNOW YOUR WORK STYLE DOSHA

Knowing more about your unique dosha can enable you to work with higher efficacy and productivity. Mainstream western culture assumes that you should start working in the morning and continue straight through until the coffee break or lunch. While some people are best suited to this approach to working, it doesn't suit all. Vata types tend to work in sprints of high productivity and then need a rest, followed by another burst of work.

Vata types ignore their disposition and body signals to their detriment. Refusing to mellow after a work sprint and pushing at high levels of productivity for long periods creates high stress and diminishing returns. Creativity burns up.

## MORNING WORK BREAK

Are you kind to your body? Do you listen, respond, and anticipate its needs? Few people treat their body with loving respect. About everyone would appreciate more energy and vitality. Who

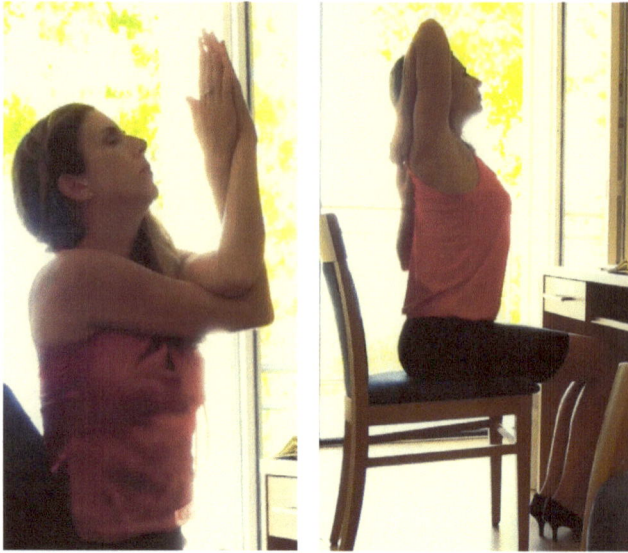

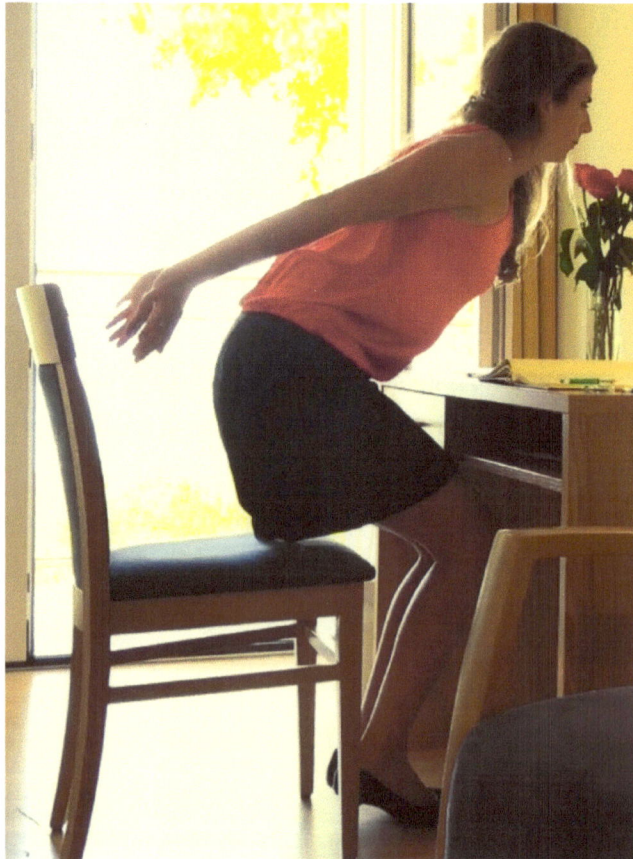

doesn't want to float through life feeling vibrant and good in their bodies while radiating a healthy glow? There is a misconception that an energetic and healthy person can flip the on switch in the morning and go, go, go like an energizer bunny straight on until evening. Popular culture thinks eating healthy foods, being thin, and exercise are what fuel this non-stop ride through the day. Most people think you need to sweat it out for at least half an hour each day to earn that high energy, health, and well-being. They're wrong. There are thin people eating only healthy foods who are exhausted and burnt out. Some more voluptuous people glow with well-being and energy. What does this mean?

If you aren't at your goal body weight or image, you don't need to wait until you shed the pounds or get fit to start feeling a rush of wellness and energy in your body. Well-being and vitality are just a few days away from listening to your body and treating it with kindness. Each body is unique, but everybody needs work breaks that replenish. If your work has you sitting in a chair for hours, then the best work break involves movement to activate your muscles and stretch. Five to ten minutes of Yoga mid-morning will refortify your energy and well-being. Free Yoga Desk videos available on Youtube at: shorturl.at/jmJ13.

Do you work in a space that inhibits you from standing up and flowing through Yoga poses? A few minutes of Yoga at your desk is the answer. Remember as a desk worker to also stand up once each hour while you check your progress against your intention.

If your work has you on your feet or working physically, then you are best served by rest for a few minutes. Optimally, you would find a place where you could lay down flat on the floor on your back for two to ten minutes. Close your eyes, place your hands on your belly, and focus on your breath. If this isn't possible, then finding a quiet place to sit with a tall spine and concentrate on your breathing will rejuvenate you.

*"Those that work without ego are extraordinarily successful at what they do." - Eckhart Tolle*

## EATING WELL ~ FUEL YOUR WORK DAY

Packing your lunch not only ensures you eat a meal low in sugar and salt and high in nutrients. It will also save you money. Chefs have a multitude of inspiring and delicious, healthy recipes you can experiment with preparing to take with you to work.

Go for a five to ten-minute walk around the block after lunch. Getting out into natural light will boost your mood and walking will stimulate and improve your digestion. Walking a few minutes after lunch outside will also dramatically improve your ability to fall asleep at night and the quality of your slumber.

### Whole Grain & Veggies Bowl
Eat 2-4 different kinds of fresh, raw veggies cut up or shredded, such as cabbage, red peppers, one cup of rice, roasted vegetables, chickpeas, or whole grain, such as bulgar, couscous, lentils and fresh herbs, such as cilantro, chives, lemon grass, dill, thyme, or basil or drizzle a green sauce on top.

### Veggie Sandwich
Wholegrain bread, sliced mozzarella layered with tomato slices, drizzled with olive oil and vinegar and fresh basil added on top to garnish.

## Berries & Oatmeal

Bring a cup of whole grain oatmeal and a cup of water to a boil. Reduce the heat to low and let simmer for 2-5 minutes until soft.

Add a half cup of fresh or frozen berries. Place in a glass container and wait until cool before placing it in the fridge for the next day or taking with you immediately to work. Sweeten with maple syrup or no sugar-added jam.

## Snacks

Bring healthy snacks with you to work to fuel your body with what it needs to thrive. A handful of walnuts, almonds, cashews, pumpkin seeds, or sunflower seeds are an excellent snack combined with a piece of fresh fruit.

Create pre-measured snack packs of nuts for the week on Sunday. Alternate the type of fruit you bring with you to work. Place two liters of pure water or a pot of unsweetened tea on your desk and drink throughout the day. Staying adequately hydrated satiates hunger, improves energy levels, and the ability to focus.

Would you like a sweet treat after lunch or in the afternoon? Baking your sweet treats yourself will enable you to reduce the quantity of sugar drastically. You may miss the sweetness at first, but you will become accustomed to the new level of sweet with time. The magic is to add spices such as cinnamon, nutmeg, and cardamom or high-quality vanilla bean to reduce the dependency on sugar. High quality pure, unsweetened cocoa can also make delicious desserts that require less sugar. Bananas, applesauce, and maple syrup can be used as sugar substitutes.

## Apple Strudel Cups

Peel and slice two apples and add to a bowl. Squeeze in the juice of half an orange. Optional: Add one tablespoon of sugar. Mix the apples with 2 teaspoons of cinnamon and Cardamom and 1 teaspoon of nutmeg. Place in muffin cups and bake at 180 degrees Celsius for 15-20 minutes, or until soft.

## STRESS MANAGEMENT: QUICK CALM

Work can be stressful. Deadlines, customers, colleagues, your children melting down, or the unexpected project that lands on your lap can trigger the stress response in the body. Your body tenses, your heart begins to race, your breath quickens and becomes shallow, and your mind races. The urge to run, fight, freeze or power through without a break can seize hold of you. Don't let stress overpower you. Set aside five minutes to turn the stress response in your body to off before responding, acting, or proceeding. Place one hand on your belly and the other over your heart. Breathe in through the nose down into your belly, up into your ribs, your side waist, and then your heart. Now breathe out through pursed lips as smoothly and slowly as you can, like a balloon ever so slowly deflating. Aim to make your exhale twice as long as your inhale, which will calm your body and mind. Repeat five times.

If you can go to a space to be alone, then the next step is to stand up tall, stacking shoulders over hips, hips over ankles. Breathe in deeply as you did before and reach your arms out and up.

As you exhale as smoothly and slowly as you can through pursed lips, begin to shake your hands slowly down towards your sides. Repeat five times. Linking breath with movement will pull you back into your body and start to release you from the stress response. Shaking the hands on the exhalation releases anxious energy and tension.

To release stress from your energy field you can place one palm over your forehead and the other over the back of your head. Breathe in deeply through the nose to the count of four and out as slowly as you can to the count of ten.

Another option is to take your fingertips to the center of your forehead, to your third eye, and place your thumbs on your temples. Gently pull the fingers toward your thumbs. Breathe deeply.

Is someone standing in front of you, provoking the stress response in your body? Is it impossible to step away for a moment? Then don't be afraid to say, "let me think for a moment," and take time for one deep, long breath and one exhale as twice as long as your inhalation. Or two breaths even. Next, smile and respond to the situation.

## 3 MINUTES - NADI SHODHANA

Sit or stand with a tall spine, stacking your shoulders directly over your hips. Take a deep breath in through your nose, expanding your belly, low lungs, and feeling your chest rise. Gently place your right thumb over your right nostril and exhale through the left. Inhale smoothly and slowly through the left nostril, then depress the left nostril with the third, ring finger and exhale out the right nostril. Inhale deeply through the right nostril, slowly expanding into all four corners of your torso. Gently close the right nostril with the right thumb and breathe out the left nostril. Continue this pattern of breathing for three minutes.

Finish your breathing practice by breathing out the left nostril, if you want to feel calmer. If you are feeling lethargic, tired, and passive, finish Nadi Shodhana by breathing out the right nostril to activate energy. Alternate nostril breathing, known as Nadi Shodhana in Sanskrit, cleanses the subtle energy of the body.

Nadi Shodhana can enable you to turn off the stress response in the body. Nadi shodhana can also strengthen your lungs and re-balance the two sides of your brain for improved focus.

## AFTERNOON ENERGY ACTIVATION

Leveraging your morning hours for creative, productive projects means you need to shift meetings, miscellaneous tasks, social media engagement, and email to the afternoon. Energy begins to wane for most people in the late afternoon. Stress can seize the body and mind caused by co-workers, customers, or the unexpected impeding work progress. Stress at work can peak in the afternoon as energy drops, and the clock counts down. Going into the flight, fight, or freeze mode inhibits perspective, cre-

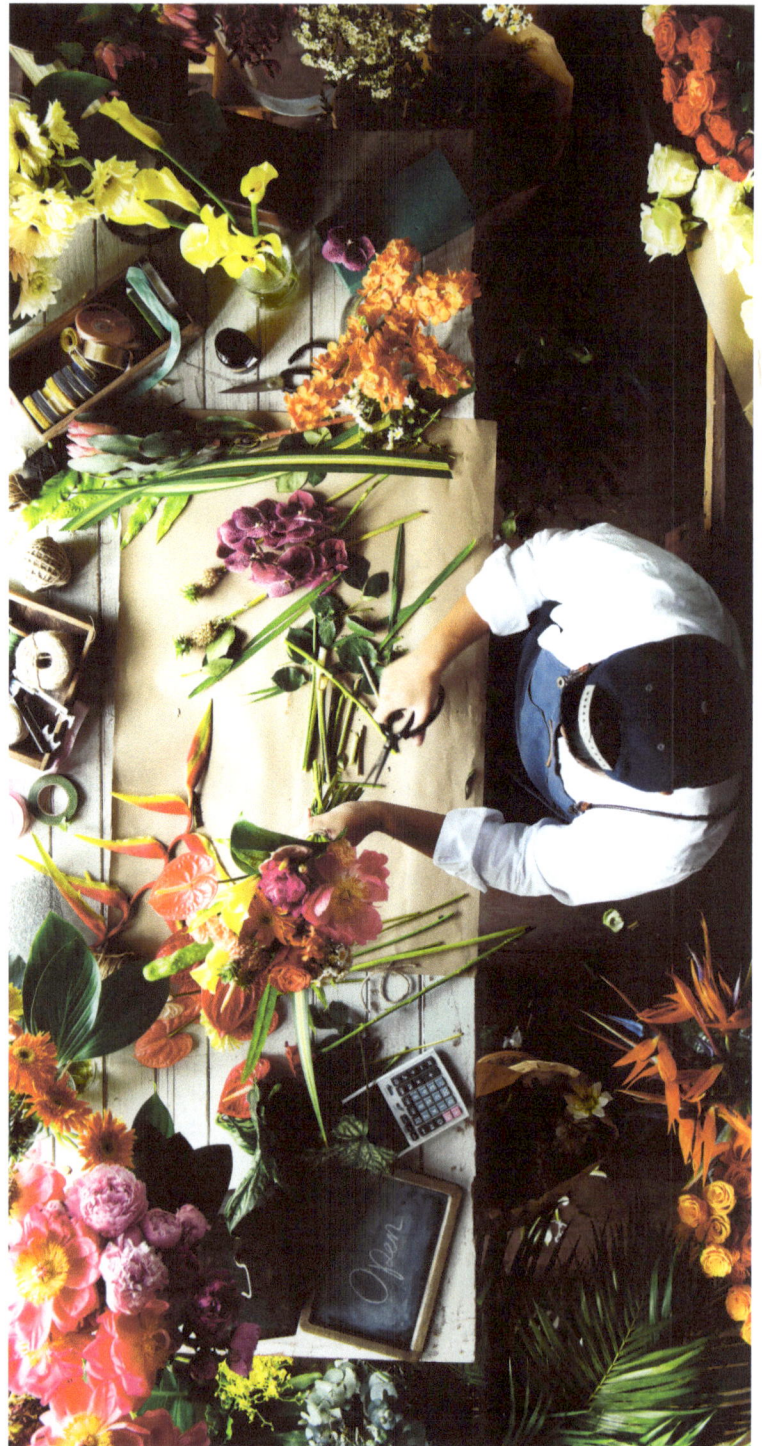

ativity, and inspiration. You may be someone who uses the rush of stress in the body to power forward through the rest of the workday. Yet it is unlikely your work will be inspired, visionary, or fulfilling while stressed.

An engine red danger sign is flashing for you if you work in a state of stress day in and day out. Chronic stress wreaks havoc on the body, mind, and soul. People and situations are different, so it is impossible to say exactly when your body will burn through all your stress hormones. The nervous system needs time to replenish itself and alternates in a healthy situation naturally between the sympathetic and parasympathetic nervous systems. If your nervous system is predominately in the stress, sympathetic status, then you become unbalanced.

There is not enough time for the body to flip on the parasympathetic state of relaxation, replenishment, and repair. Once you use up all your stress hormones, your body will compensate with sex hormones until those are depleted as well. The final station is a state of burn out.

You don't need to book a spa weekend or travel to a tropical beach every few weeks to rejuvenate. Attention and kindness to your body throughout the work day will keep replenishing you with energy and wellness.

Notice when stress creeps up on you at work. Do your shoulders tense up by your ears? Your breathing becomes shallow? Your posture hunched? Your solar plexus or stomach clenched?

Once you notice the signals of stress in your body, take a two to five-minute break. Reconnect and deepen the breath. Bring your hand to your belly and heart. Expand the breath up your torso on the inhalation, and relax your shoulders down away from your ears on the exhalation. You can lower the hormones cortisol, norepinephrine, epinephrine, and catecholamines while raising the feel-good hormones serotonin, dopamine, and oxytocin through self-massage, aromatherapy, and linking breath with movement.

Taking a few minutes to engage in breath work and link breath with movement can boost your well-being in minutes. Add some Yoga into your workday.

For a quick energy activation you can place your right hand on your left shoulder and draw it across your body to your left hip. Bring your left hand to the right shoulder and draw across your body to your left hip. Repeat three to five times while expanding the breath into the belly, low ribs, and heart and breathing out as slowly as you can. Visit Yoga Desk - Yoga with Heather on YouTube for more Yoga flows you can do at your desk in two to ten minutes to quickly melt away stress, increase your suppleness, and improve your creativity and concentration. To fortify yourself against stress and boost resilience bathe in nature regularly and go walking daily. Go for a

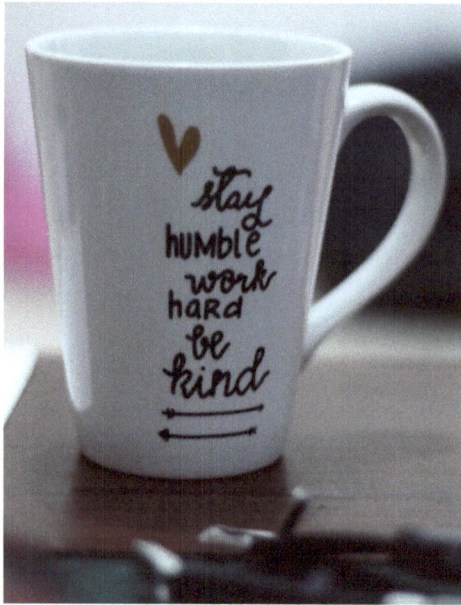

"If you can't do great things, do little things with great love. If you can't do them with great love, do them with a little love. If you can't do them with a little love, do them anyway." - Mother Teresa

"The opposite of fear is love - love of the challenge, love of the work, the pure joyous passion to take a shot at our dream and see if we can pull it off."
- Steven Pressfield

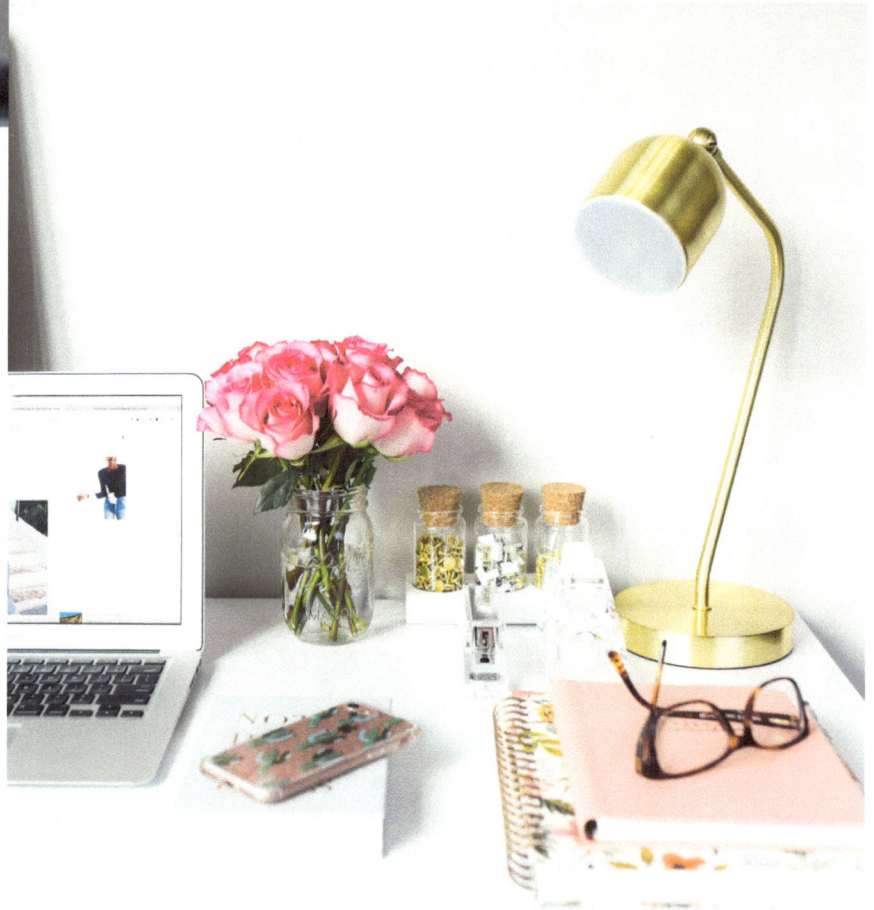

walk everyday for fifteen to thirty minutes and no matter what the weather. Spend time in nature daily or looking at green to reduce stress while boosting your vitality and mood. Turn spending time walking into a habit by going the same time everyday: as soon as you get home from work, after you eat lunch, or right after dinner.

## ACUPRESSURE TO DESTRESS & ENERGIZE

**Third Eye.** Your third eye is located in the middle of your forehead. Press your third eye with your fingers for fifteen seconds, release, then repeat five times to soothe stress.

**Sea of tranquility.** The "Sea of Tranquility" is found in the middle of the sternum, the bone running down the middle of the chest. To find the exact pressure point, press your fingers to the middle of the sternum. Press the "Sea of Tranquility" point for thirty seconds to two minutes to release stress, tension, anxiety, and emotional turmoil.

**Spirit Gate.** Take your thumb and trace it down your little finger, across the palm, to your wrist crease. Press this pressure point on the wrist directly below the little finger, called the "Spirit Gate," for thirty seconds to relax, re-balance, and refresh. Finish by rubbing your palms together and then cupping them over the eyes.

**Palm Point.** Calm your entire body by firmly pressing your thumb into the palm of your hand. Breathe in and out slowly and smoothly through the nose three times. Then circle your thumb in the center of your palm while still applying pressure for three long, slow breaths in and out the nose. Switch directions and rotate the thumb in the other direction for three breaths. Repeat on the opposite palm. Finish by rubbing your palms together and resting them over the solar plexus for three breaths.

**Sea of Vitality.** Find the "Sea of Vitality" point by cinching your waist with your hands. Next, slide your palms up your side body until your thumbs feel the lowest ribs on your back. Press your thumbs just below your last ribs on either side of your spine for two long, slow, deep belly breaths in and out the nose. Glide your thumbs two finger widths away from the spine and press the thumbs into the back for two breaths. Repeat twice to increase your energy.

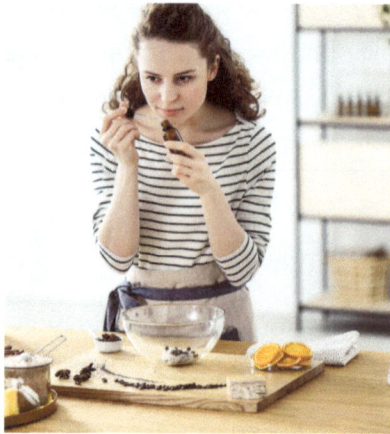
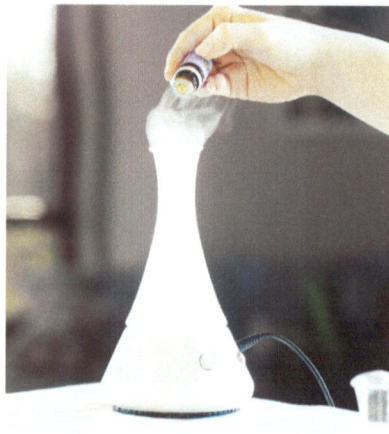
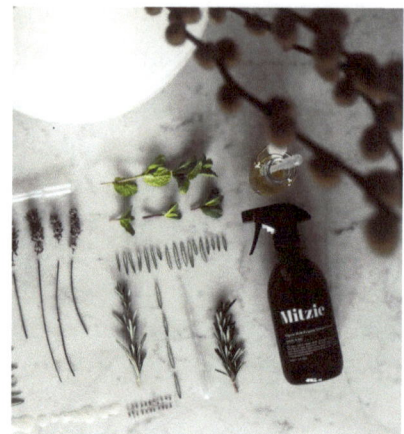

## AROMATHERAPY AT WORK

You could be lucky enough to be able to introduce an essential oil diffuser to your place of work. If not, you can still leverage aromatherapy at work to stimulate stress-relief, energize, uplift, or focus. You can inhale the scent direct from the bottle, or you can take a cloth handkerchief or cut an old t-shirt into squares. Sprinkle two to four drops of essential oil onto the cloth square and raise to just below your chin. Breathe slowly and deeply in and out your nose for one to three minutes to inhale the benefits of the scent. Do not allow the undiluted essential oil to come in contact with your skin.

Essential oils are the concentrated extracts of plants and will cause skin irritation, burning, or worse if used on the skin undiluted. Always mix essential oils with a carrier oil. Excellent carrier oils are olive, jojoba, sweet almond, sunflower seed, avocado, and grape seed. Add six essential oil drops to one ounce of carrier oil to dilute them safely for use. Another option is to add six drops of essential oil to one ounce of water in a mist bottle.

Mist the spray on your face to destress or uplift. Explore your reaction to the scent of different essential oils and oil blends and their effect on your mood, energy, ability to focus, anxiety, and stress levels. While some love citrus oils, others prefer the warm, spicy scents. You may find the citrus scents lift your spirits or that you prefer spicy, exotic scents.

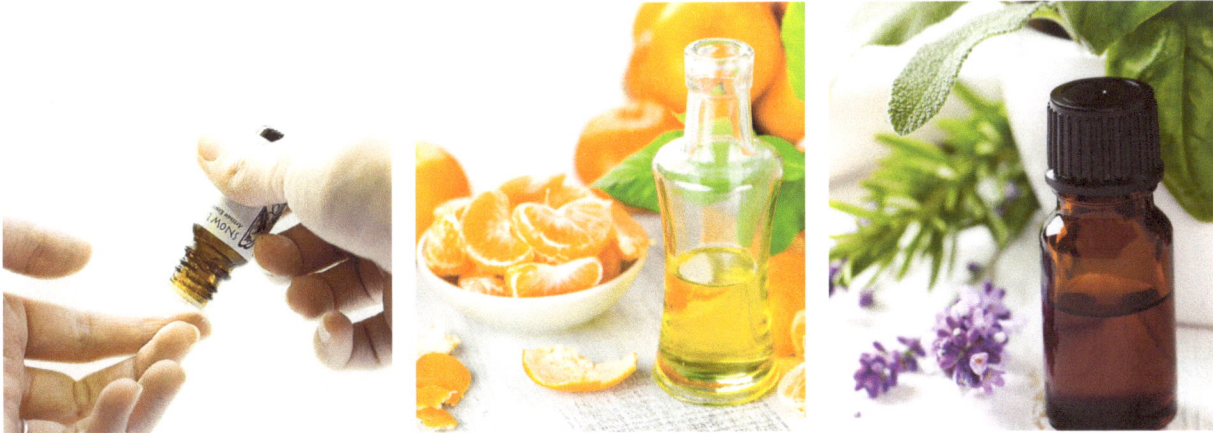

## SCENTS TO UPLIFT, IMPROVE FOCUS, ENERGIZE

**LEMON:** A scientific study reported that smelling lemon oil caused the participants' moods to improve and norepinephrine, a hormone that reduces stress, lowered in their bloodstream.

**ORANGE:** The scent of orange oil is balancing and uplifting to mind and mood.

**LIME:** Lime essential oil is both uplifting and energizing.

**GRAPEFRUIT:** Grapefruit essential oil boosts mood and balances emotions.

**FRANKINCENSE:** Counteracts depression and anxiety. Frankincense lifts your energy levels and concentration.

**YLANG YLANG:** Ylang ylang expands the heart and works like a natural anti-depressant.

**GINGER:** Ginger essential oil works to revitalize your energy levels and mood.

**CINNAMON:** Cinnamon essential oil can give you an energy boost when you're feeling sluggish.

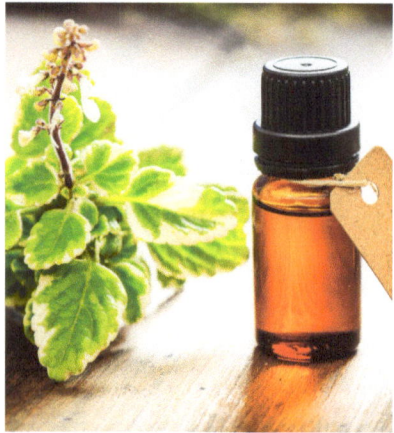

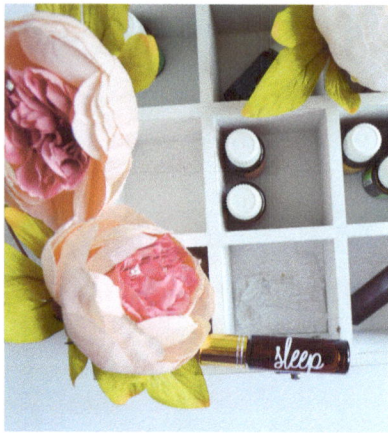

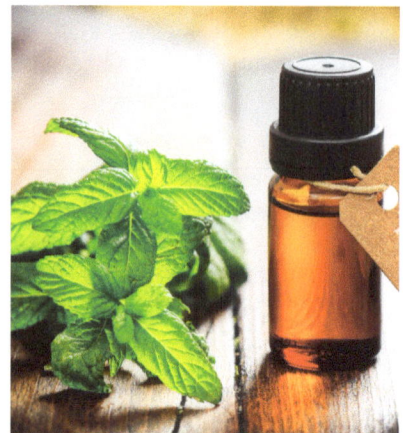

## SCENTS TO INCREASE ENERGY & CONCENTRATION

**EUCALYPTUS & PEPPERMINT OIL:** Feeling exhausted? Add a few drops of eucalyptus or peppermint oil to a diffuser, your misting bottle, or lotion and inhale to stimulate the mind and body. Peppermint can wake you up and improve your ability to concentrate and retain information.

## UNWIND & DESTRESS SCENTS

**CEDAR WOOD & LAVENDER OIL:** Lavender is not only relaxing, but also anti-anxiety, anti-inflammatory, antimicrobial, antiviral, antibacterial, and even immune-boosting. Cedar wood can boost your production of serotonin white; it reduces tension and stress.

## STRESS RELIEF BLEND
- 3 drops lavender, 3 drops frankincense
- 1 drop ylang-ylang, 2 drops cedar wood, 3 drops lavender, 2 drops orange

## ENERGY & FOCUS BLENDS
- 4 drops orange, 4 drops peppermint
- 2 drops cinnamon, 3 drops orange,
3 drops frankincense

## UPLIFT BLENDS
- 3 drops orange, 3 drops lime, 3 drops lavender
- 2 drops grapefruit, 2 drops peppermint

## WORK DAY END

You can end your workday by clearing and cleaning your desk and laptop. Organize and file all paper and electronic files. Do a quick sweep to ensure your desk and workspace only has elements that spark joy or are necessary for future work.

Take a few minutes at the end of the day to evaluate your day's progress against short, medium, and long-term project goals. Did you hit your targets for the day? If not, what impeded your efforts? Brainstorm a way to make up for the lack of progress the next day. Perhaps coming into the office an hour earlier, or clearing an entire evening to work late will allow you to enter a state of flow.

Falling away from the world around you and releasing all sense of time can enable you to glide through work and achieve measurable progress.

Motivation, energy, and productivity will return once you have surged forward in the project and escaped the stress-inducing claws of time pressure.

*"Resistance is the response of the frightened, petty, small-time ego to the brave, generous, magnificent impulse of the creative self." - Steven Pressfield*

## WORK FENG SHUI

A desk and workspace with dynamic and tranquil energy instills concentration and creativity. Vibrant colors, nature, open white space, soothing sounds, and soft clothing against the skin promote well-being and joy. Unfortunately, most workspaces are predominated by shades of gray.

Add vitality and wellness to your desk by opening up blank space on your desk. Stimulate good energy to flow at your desk and in the room where you work by clearing away all clutter. Analyze every object on and in your office using the Konmari method.

Hold the paper, book, or miscellaneous object in your hand, and feel whether it sparks joy. Only keep things that spark joy visible on your desk. Some elements may not spark joy, but be something you want or need to take with you into your future to achieve your goals. Organize these belongings in files, folders, and in small boxes of various sizes, so they fit neatly in your drawers and on your shelves. Once you are organized and only have elements that spark joy on your desk, it's time to add a dash of color. A bowl of oranges, lemons, limes, or a mixture of fruit adds a stroke of hue to your desk. A vase of fresh flowers stimulates your office with fresh energy and color. A cup of tree branches creates texture and brings the green of the outdoors inside. A bowl or vase of crystals sparkle with light. You may be fortunate enough to work in a space which allows you to introduce a desk water fountain. The movement of the water stirs up positive energy as the sound calms.

## WORK DAY PRODUCTIVITY & RESULTS

Do you want to triumph in your work and achieve results? Are you ready to vanquish what is stealing your time and energy? Is it time to stop struggling, grow a backbone, and reach higher levels of productivity? Read on to find out what prolific superstars do every day to unleash their success and wellness.

### 1.   Set Audacious Goals

Don't just set audacious goals, write them down. Refer to the goals every morning. Research someone who has achieved what you desire and use their path as a guide. Visualize the steps and actions you need to take to get to where you want to go. Big and brave goals will release energy. Most importantly: go and take ACTION towards achieving the goals every day.

### 2.   Join the 5 am Club

Some of the healthiest and most successful people on the planet wake up early every morning. Wake up at five, and you're earning yourself two to three hours to invest in exercise, self-care, learning, and working without distraction or interruptions. Start getting up every morning at five to start your day. Does this sound impossible? Prime your mind at night before you fall asleep. Promise

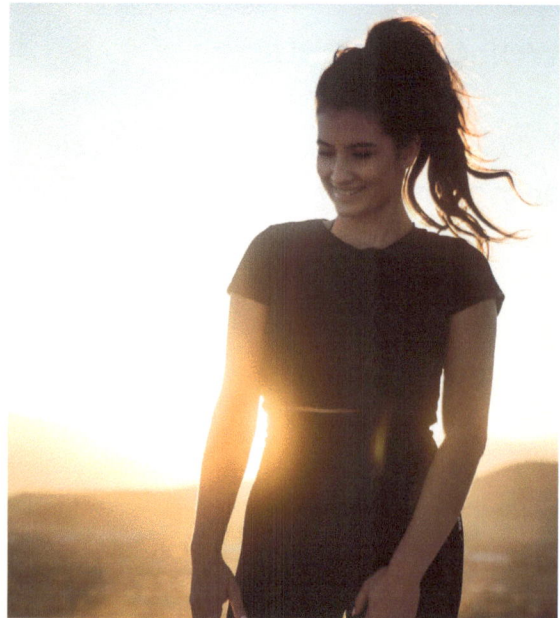

yourself that the second you open your eyes, you will count to three and jump out of bed. It sounds stupid. It will work after 41 days, which is how long we need to imprint a habit.

### 3.   Start Your Day with Yoga & Meditation

You may know that yoga and meditation have a long list of benefits for your health. Did you know that Yoga will improve your productivity too?

Commit to starting your day each morning with Yoga, and you will be training your mind to focus. Focusing on the breath and tuning in to the observer within you will pull your attention away from mindless thought loops and being emotionally reactive. You won't just get more productive. You'll start devoting your best energy to the work that matters the most.

### 4.   GO! Immediate Action

Stop thinking and start acting. Count to three and act. Speak out your innovative idea at the meeting. Create a new video. Call up the potential client. Action will create a feedback loop that will positively fuel more activity. You don't get work done by thinking about the possibilities.

### 5.   Stay Active All Day

The ultimate productivity tool in the world is exercise. So do some early morning Yoga at five am, then go for a walk after lunch, or engage in aerobic or strengthening exercise in the evening.

Stand up at least once every sixty minutes to move. Go outside, climb some stairs, do some desk yoga, or get old school and do twenty jumping jacks. The movement will boost your energy, sharpen your focus, and enable you to sit down to work again refreshed.

### 6.   Your Best Physical Fitness

Strive towards reaching the best physical fitness of your life to watch your energy explode.

### 7.   Iron Routines

What do Thomas Edison, Stephen King, and John Grisham have in common? They are all successful in their careers and masters of productivity, and they follow strict routines. Their routine regulates everything from when they get up in the morning, to when they work, exercise, and relax. Create a routine and stick to it to maximize your mastery and productivity.

## 8.  Be a Minimalist

Dirt and clutter suck the energy out of a room and infringe on your productivity and creativity. De-clutter your office, home, car, schedule, and relationships. Simplify and streamline. Do you need all those apps on your phone? Is your productivity app saving you time, or wasting it? Delete it! Go for clean, empty spaces to free your brain to produce its most brilliant work in record time.

## 9.  Be Consistent

Invest time every day in working on the medium and long-term projects that are most critical to the success of your career or business. Even ten minutes a day adds up to over an hour each week. Don't underestimate the power of showing up and investing the time every single day.

## 10.  Eat That Frog

Set a priority at the close of every workday for the next day. Get your most critical work done before lunch the next day.

## 11.  Eliminate the Energy Vampires

Eliminate the energy vampires from your life that are sucking away your excitement, enthusiasm, and self-belief. If you can't eliminate energy vampires, take immediate action to counterbalance them with people, activities, and media that will cause your motivation to soar.

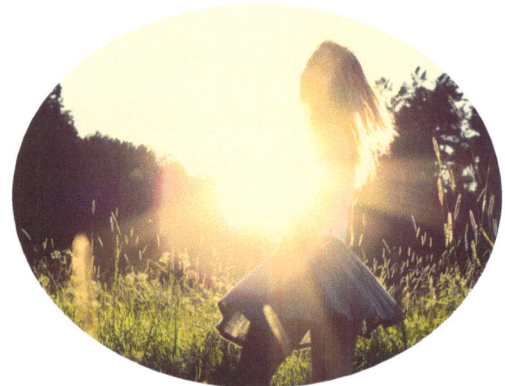

## 12.  Seek Out Inspiration & Positive Energy

You are going after audacious goals. You need positive energy to spiral you upwards. Be aware of everyone and everything that influences you in your life.

Actively seek out podcasts, books, documentaries, people, groups, and activities that inspire, motivate, and charge you with energy to act.

## 13.  5 Minute Rule

Do it now if it will take five minutes or less instead of putting it on a list or wasting mind space

UNLESS you are in your flow of pure focus in the morning on your critical work. Don't let anything pull your attention away from what matters the most, even for five minutes. Give anyone also the courtesy of five minutes. At the end of five minutes explain how you will take action or follow-up with them at a later date.

## 14. Release Addictions

You can sell your TV, ban all news sites from your laptop and phone, commit to living drama free from this moment forward, ban all excessive alcohol, drugs, and sugar consumption, give-up complaining, exit the lousy relationship, refrain from gossip, or stop shopping. Release what is stealing your energy.

## 15. Work in Batches

Schedule similar tasks to be done in one focused session. Do not do one video for your You-tube channel. Spend a day getting eight videos done for the entire month. Do not create one podcast. Schedule a day to complete four all at once. Instead of visiting one client, schedule meetings with five on the same day.

## 16. Primary Consistent Focus

What is the ONE THING that is the critical key to your future success and growth in your career or business? Dedicate time each day to this main thing in the morning. Set goals and seek out learning and mentoring to improve your mastery of your ONE THING.

## 17. Laser Your Focus

Do not multi-task. Stop the leap from one task to the next. Spend a few hours each day working on one activity. You will gain scales of economy as your mind, body, and attention flow into the work. Don't be surprised if you get even double the work done.

## 18. Hide for a Few Hours Daily

Do you get your best work done in the office? Hide for a few hours each day to escape all interruptions and distractions so you can achieve pure focus. Devote your full attention to producing flawless, highly innovative or creative work.

## 19. Write a NO List

Do you have a to-do list? You need a NO-LIST even more. Brainstorm all the activities that are using up time and energy and preventing you from making leaps forward to your professional and personal success. Commit to eliminating everything on your NO-LIST from your life.

## 20. Disciplined Daydreaming

Unleash the vibrant potential of your creativity and innovation by letting your subconscious process and integrate. Before the digital world people had time to think while they waited in lines, for trains, while walking, while waiting in a restaurant for friends to appear. To kick ass at work and be the most productive person you know you need to schedule the time to sit and think. Allocating time to disciplined daydreaming will enable you to make connections, find new inspiration, or clear your brain of thoughts and focus on mindfulness and the present moment.

## 21. Does it Thrill You? Say Yes

Start only saying yes to what thrills you. Otherwise, say no, find a way to outsource the work, or minimize the amount of time and energy you must invest.

## 22. Double Your Learning Rate

What are you working on learning right now? What book are you reading? What course are you attending? To boost your productivity you need to be learning every day. Either sign up for a class, or put together your own curriculum of books, podcasts, audio books and articles to learn and master the area that will kick your career, business, or personal growth into high-gear.

## 23. Schedule Time for Rejuvenation

Take time to replenish and nourish your body, mind, and soul daily, weekly and each season. Retreat yourself. A rested and refreshed body and mind will accelerate your career when you turn your attention back to your work.

## 24. Not Everyone Needs to Like You

You need to get comfortable with people not liking you to become the most productive person you know. Do you want to supercharge your productivity and accomplish your goals? You can't say yes to every request.

Most of us have an intrinsic need to be liked, so we say yes to everything. You can Stop.

## 25.   Outsource What You Hate
You don't need to do work you hate.. You can outsource work and save your willpower.

## 26.   Build Your Influence
Build your influence by adding value to peoples' lives. Help others to grow or achieve their goals and dreams. Pro-actively contribute to the community.

## 27.   Know Your Strengths. Continually Improve
What are your top three character strengths, technical strengths, and knowledge strengths? Know where you are strong and what you enjoy doing the most. Play to your strengths and invest time every day in continually improving your mastery in your top three in each area.

*"The ego tends to equate having with Being: I have, therefore I am. And the more I have, the more I am. The ego lives through comparison."- Eckhart Tolle*

*"It's not enough to yearn for more in your life. Your desire must be specific; it must point from where you are to where you want to be." - Deepak Chopra*

*"Everyone has his own specific vocation or mission in life to carry out a concrete assignment which demands fulfillment. Therein he cannot be replaced, nor can his life be repeated." - Viktor E. Frankl*

You can release the craving and striving for more belongings, money, prestige, and admiration in the eyes of others. Move from the place of the soul. Find the meaning of your life, not once, but over and over again. Let your life purpose  and values define your goals, guide your actions, and color the design of your life from a place of quiet stillness.

# Financial, Career, Home Wellness Evaluation & Affirmations

| | Highly disagree | Disagree | Slightly disagree | Slightly agree | Agree | Strongly agree |
|---|---|---|---|---|---|---|
| I know how much money I would like to be making 5 years from now. | | | | | | |
| I manage my money well. | | | | | | |
| I seldom experience financial stress. | | | | | | |
| I have clear, written financial goals. | | | | | | |
| I deeply understand the fundamentals of wealth creation. | | | | | | |
| I believe that making money and creating wealth are very good things. | | | | | | |
| My finances are highly organized. | | | | | | |
| My personal business life is highly organized (insurance, estate plan, etc.). | | | | | | |
| I have a high level of financial security in my life. | | | | | | |
| I have thought deeply about my career and know exactly what I want in this area of my life. | | | | | | |
| I currently have a plan in place for achieving my ideal life. | | | | | | |
| I feel confident and proud of the work I do most of the time. | | | | | | |
| I feel vibrant, balanced, and content at work. | | | | | | |
| I can clearly define my single most important     goal in life. | | | | | | |
| My career is very fulfilling to me. I love what I do. | | | | | | |
| I find my career challenges me and keeps me learning and growing. | | | | | | |
| I seldom experience stress at work. | | | | | | |

| | Highly disagree | Disagree | Slightly disagree | Slightly agree | Agree | Strongly agree |
|---|---|---|---|---|---|---|
| • I wake up each morning looking forward to my work. | | | | | | |
| • I am very good at what I do. | | | | | | |
| • I do not wish to change my job. | | | | | | |
| • I am more than my job, finances, home, city, belongings. | | | | | | |
| • I love the place where I live. | | | | | | |
| • I have turned where I live into a home. | | | | | | |
| • My home inspires the emotions I want us to feel, like serenity, coziness, luxury, fun. | | | | | | |
| • My home is clean. | | | | | | |
| • My home is organized. | | | | | | |
| • My home contains belongings that spark joy. | | | | | | |
| • I take time to make nourishing, nutritious meals the majority of the time. | | | | | | |
| • I am proud of my home. | | | | | | |

# Intellectual & Physical Wellness Evaluation & Affirmations

| | Highly disagree | Disagree | Slightly disagree | Slightly agree | Agree | Strongly agree |
|---|---|---|---|---|---|---|
| I believe in and pursue life long learning and personal development. | | | | | | |
| I feel fulfilled intellectually. | | | | | | |
| I have a plan in place to keep myself learning and my mind growing. | | | | | | |
| I believe that if you don't use it, you start to lose it. | | | | | | |
| I push myself mentally and grow my intellectual abilities daily through active learning. | | | | | | |
| I am happy with my current weight. | | | | | | |
| I don't smoke. | | | | | | |
| I don't drink more than a glass of alcohol per day. | | | | | | |
| I feel beautiful or attractive. | | | | | | |
| I am very happy with the way my body looks. | | | | | | |
| I have thought about my health and fitness and know exactly what I want. | | | | | | |
| I have a clearly defined exercise routine and I stick to it. | | | | | | |
| I have an nutritious, healthy diet. | | | | | | |
| I am very happy with the way I feel inside my body. | | | | | | |
| I have educated myself regarding health and nutrition. | | | | | | |
| I look and feel younger than my true age. | | | | | | |
| I have a consistently high energy level. | | | | | | |
| I take time for self-care and my appearance. | | | | | | |

# Homemaking

*"Spread love everywhere you go; first of all in your house. Give love to your children, to your wife or husband, to a next door neighbor. Let no one ever come to you without leaving better and happier." - Mother Teresa*

Whether you live alone, with friends, or with a family, making a home out of where you live can infuse your life with more wellness. Waking up in a place which feels safe, cozy, beautiful, or uplifting increases your life quality. Being able to return to a safe haven after being out in the world is a source of satisfaction and strength. Turning where you live into a home is an art and requires work. Unfortunately in modern society, only compensated work is esteemed. Unpaid work, such as homemaking, is deemed of lesser esteem than bringing in a paycheck.

Your values and your outlook belong to you. You are free to change your mind and see the world with new eyes whenever you want.

Few people enjoy cleaning and see it as a necessary activity to get done. You can try seeing cleaning and chores as all part of the art of homemaking. Making a home for yourself and for others is a gift of wellness. Create an environment you love filled with textures, scents, sounds, and colors that spark calm, joy, inspiration, focus, relaxation, creativity, or well-being.

## CLEANING

The first step to creating a happy home experience is cleaning. A clean space is not only clear of dirt, dust, and grime but also free of negative energy. Cleaning sweeps the old energy away.

Habit stacking works with cleaning as well as it does with the Morning Revitalize Routine. Start your cleaning, organizing, and chores habit stacking at the same time each day, like right after dinner. Quickly flow through dishes, vacuuming, doing a quick clean of the bathrooms, and picking up and placing belongings all back in their 'homes' every day. End your homemaking flow with lighting candles, spraying an essential oil mist in each room, or turning on music to elevate the energy of the home. Placing fresh cut flowers, a bowl of vibrant colored fruit, tree branches, or a collection of crystals or stones in the kitchen and living areas brings natural energy into the home.

Every weekend set aside some time to flow through a deep clean. Almost everyone out there loves the feeling of slipping into fresh, clean sheets. Give yourself and those you love the luxury of clean linens at least once every ten days to boost well-being.

## MINIMALISM

White and blank space is relaxing for the mind, body, and spirit. Look at luxury modern interior design, and you will find clear surfaces, open spaces, and less, instead of more, furniture in a room. It doesn't matter how small the area is within which you live. You can gift yourself the luxurious feeling of more blank space.

Owning fewer belongings means there is less to keep organized and it is quicker to clean a room. Too many belongings can start to weigh us down unconsciously. It's time to lighten up with a belonging detox.

Start with your favorite room in the house. Pick up every object and pause. Does your energy get light, or heavier? Often we keep things because they were expensive, or out of guilt or nostalgia. No matter how expensive or sentimental, if your energy gets heavier when you pick something up, then it is time

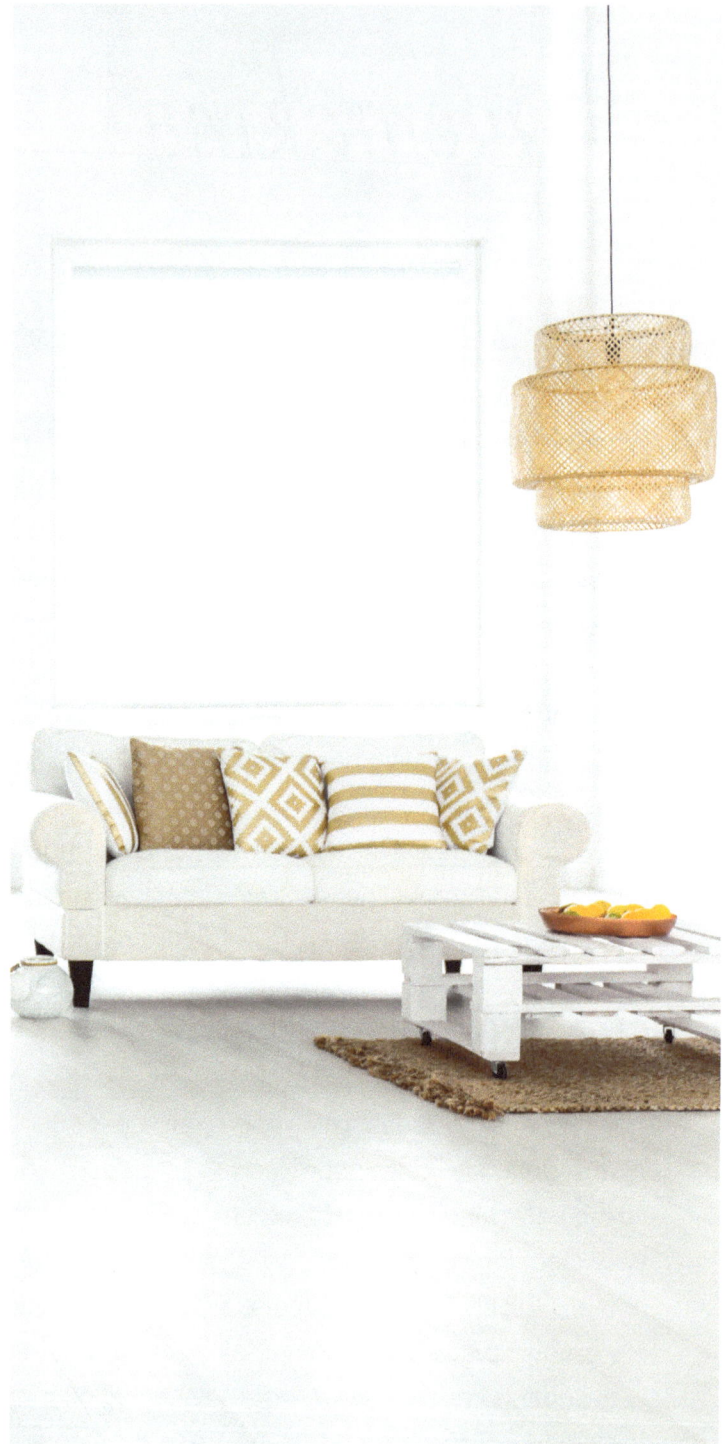

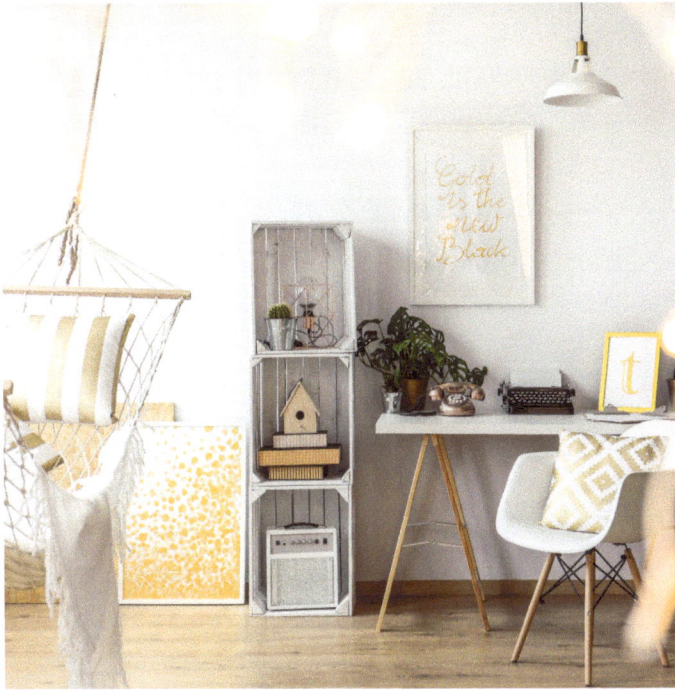

to donate, gift, or throw the item away. If you are having trouble feeling any energy when you pick things up, then start with something you know elicits joy, followed by something you know you dislike. Get in touch with what it feels like to hold these belongings, and then continue forward.

When you are done purging the room of everything that lowers your energy, then it is time to organize. Give every belonging you own a 'home.' Have a home for your keys, the mail, and a file or box for each person who lives with you to place papers, magazines, and books they are currently reading.

Use boxes to keep cords, cables, and electronics organized. Hang clothes on matching hangers sorted by color or seasonal use. If you have a dresser, then begin to fold your shirts in a way in which you can see every shirt and sweater when you open the drawer. If you have only a closet, you can do the same thing by using a box.

Fold the long outside edges of the shirt to meet in the middle, then fold the shirt over in thirds. Place the shirt 'standing' upright in the drawer. When folding towels and sheets, fold them in half, then in thirds, and then one or two more times. Stack the towels and sheets neatly one on top of the other, or you can place 'standing up' in a wicker basket and place on a shelf. Detox one room each week and finish with storage spaces and the ga-

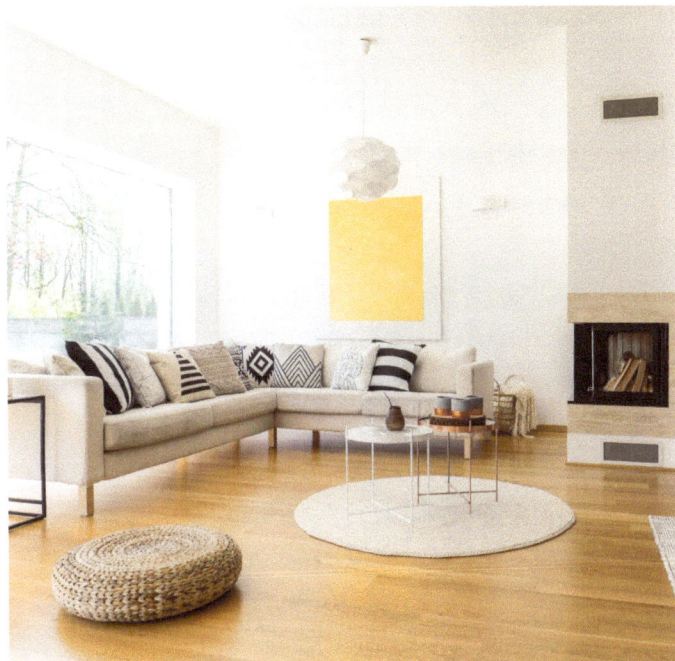

rage. Once your home is light and full of positive energy, keep it that way by being conscious of what you bring into your home. If someone gifts you something you don't want, place it in a designated storage space until you can re-gift or donate it to someone else. Being mindful while shopping and only buy something new if you are willing to gift, donate, or throw away something first to make space. Invest instead into bringing the energy of fresh cut flowers, candles, essential oils, natural bathing products, a fountain with a relaxing sound, or new music into your living space. Create a beautiful atmosphere and raise the vibrational energy of your home.

## FENG SHUI for LUXURY

How do you change your home into a luxury experience with Feng shui? Take a look at luxury homes and hotels, and a few elements become clear. There is no clutter. Everything is sparkling clean. The bedding, sheets, and towels are of high quality. There is an abundance of bright, open space and even a water feature, such as a sparkling turquoise swimming pool, or even a stream running right through the house.

Fresh cut flowers are placed not only in the living room, but also put on bedside tables and in the bathrooms. Texture is used to create contrast with smooth surfaces in the form of cushions, throw blankets, or other decorative elements. The rooms smell fresh and clean. The rooms feel balanced and inviting.

You can invite luxury and positive energy into your life no matter what your financial situation. Save up and buy the highest quality towels and sheets you can afford. Clear clutter from all surfaces and surround yourself with only things you love and raise your energy. Purge your home and life of every item that isn't necessary for eliciting joy.

Invest time into a deep clean once a week and daily cleaning to keep your home feeling luxurious. Place fresh cut flowers in bathrooms and beside the beds. Create a balanced atmosphere in living areas by rearranging furniture, so it creates a square or circle, instead of just facing a television. Place a coffee table in the middle of the furniture with a potted plant or fresh flowers and candles. Clear desks of papers and clutter and invest in sources of indirect lighting to create a relaxing, cozy, and intimate atmosphere. Use mirrors or water features in living areas to increase the sense of space or energy in a room. Add fresh potted plants, flowers, and herbs selectively to spaces to bring the positive, healing power of nature inside. Play music with a cleansing, healing frequency or nature sounds to clean the energy of your home once a day.

# Care Giving

*"If you want to change the world, go home and love your family."*
*-Mother Teresa*

## PARENTING

Do you walk around with guilt hanging on your back like a backpack filled with rocks because you aren't sure if you're a good enough parent? Does the challenge of being a good parent feel overwhelming? Are you exhausted with little time leftover for yourself? Does the day escape you and suddenly it's bedtime, and you haven't connected with your child on a deep level? You aren't alone. I feel like that sometimes too. Take some time to reflect on what kind of parent you want to be to your kids and write it down. Translate your values into action items and add them into everyday life with your kids - no matter how busy life gets.

Looking for inspiration in creating your list? Here is my day to day 'Action Sheet' for being a good parent to my children when crunched for time on busy day:

### Step 1. Ten minutes

Kids need vitamins and minerals from vegetables and fruit, whole grain-rich foods as well as lean protein. I will cut up at least four different vegetables and give them to my kids to eat before their main meal. When crunched for time during the week I will cut up the veggies and fruit on Sunday and place in Tupperware. I will buy or make whole grain (not partial whole grain; you need to read the label), bread and pasta. It takes ten minutes to cook up whole grain pasta for dinner and add a sauce. I won't feel guilty if they eat veggies, whole grain toast and scrambled eggs with ham for dinner. It may not be gourmet, but it's healthy. I will insist my kids eat some fresh cut up fruit or veggies before any other snack. I will always have plenty of fruit, nuts, veggies and whole grains in the home.

## Step 2. Twenty minutes

I will take the kids outside on a walk, a bike ride, or to the playground everyday for at least twenty minutes.

## Step 3. Ten minutes

I will learn, read, play a game, create, sing, color, dance, or just be with my child with my full attention for at least ten minutes everyday.

## Step 4. Ten Minutes

I will shower or bathe younger children, brush teeth, apply lotion in a mini massage, make sure nails are trimmed. When the kids are old enough to bathe alone I will dedicate this time to giving them a back rub, listening to music with them, or just hearing about their day. I will make sure each child will be going to bed early enough to get the 9-14 hours of sleep they need to grow and thrive.

## Step 5. Ten minutes

I will take time every day to read to each child, or cuddle and talk about the day with undivided attention, meditate, or pray. I will offer a big hug goodnight, tell them how lovable they are, and praise their effort over results. I will use this time to ask for forgiveness if I need to. If I was short-tempered or have something weighing on my conscience, now is the time I will seek resolution, so we can all go to sleep in peace.

## Things I Want to Remember as a Parent:

• Treat your kids at eye level Heather. If you wouldn't talk, treat or react to your partner or best friend in that way, then don't act that way with your child either.

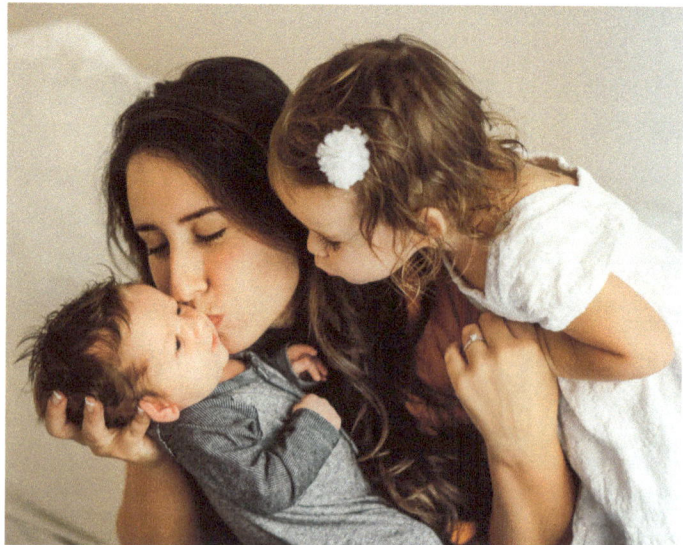

- Set boundaries. You deserve to be treated with respect. Be yourself with your kids. Say what you want and what you need. Kids respond better to your authenticity than a perfect parent role you are playing with "you should".

- Allow negative emotions to exist. How would you feel if your partner insisted you needed to be permanently happy and compliant? Yeah. Sadness, anger, jealousy, anxiety and other negative emotions are normal. Give your kids an opportunity to feel their feelings without hurting themselves or other people. Help your kids write their own joy lists for positive go-to ways to uplift and regain their balance.

- Find the joy of connection through play, laughter, dance, leaning, reading, exercise, and being in nature.

- Allow your child time to just BE. Live your own life. Role model living a beautiful life filled with joy, love, purpose, and wellness. Your actions speak louder than words ever could.

- Be patient. Practice empathy.

- It's okay to talk about what you and your kids both need and want to enjoy the time together and feel loved. Kids sense when you are spending time with them out of obligation, versus really enjoying the time in their company. Be present, be here, enjoy. Discover your kid's primary love language. Is it quality, time, gifts, acts of service, affection, or words of affirmation and support? Speak their love language.

- Dear Heather, be willing to ask for forgiveness when you can't manage to do anything on this list at all. Older children can jump in for you if you are sick or aren't available and make some of the list for younger children. Regain your wellness, balance, and priorities, and start living your good parent values again as soon as you can :)

Now it's YOUR TURN to reflect on YOUR VALUES and what good parents habits you want to incorporate into your daily life. Allocate a specific amount of time to each activity and commit to doing it everyday. Wishing you inner peace and strength as you raise your healthy, conscious, and joyful child!

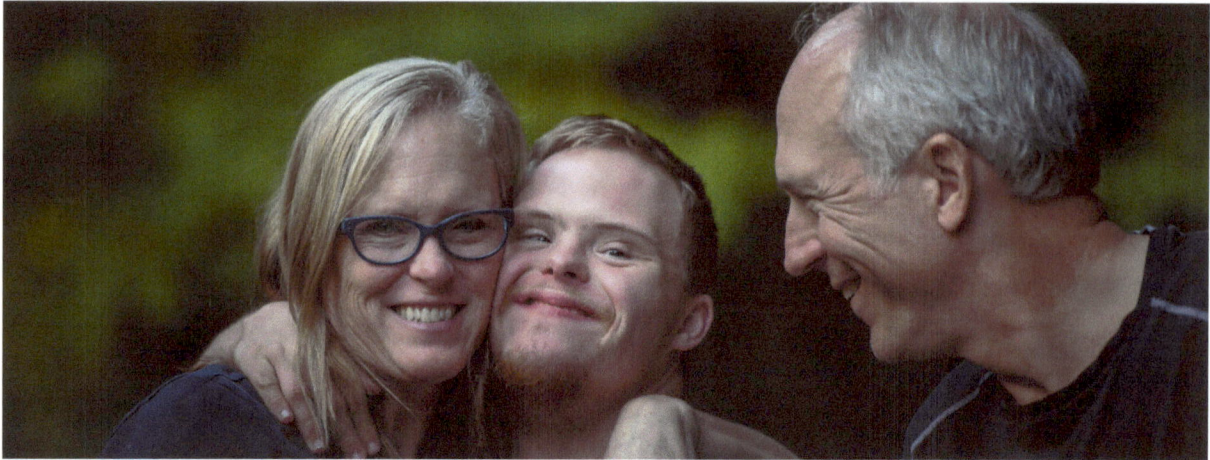
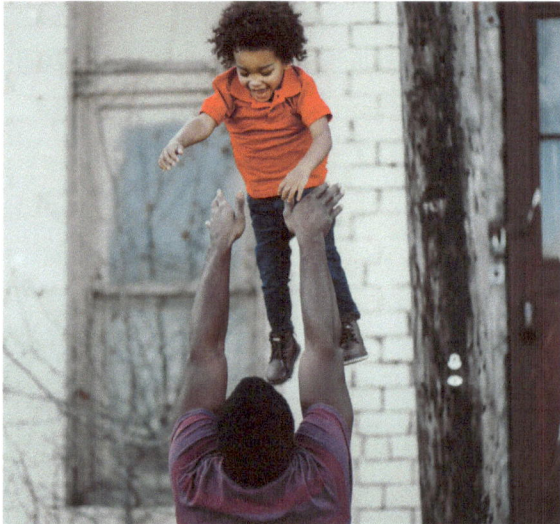
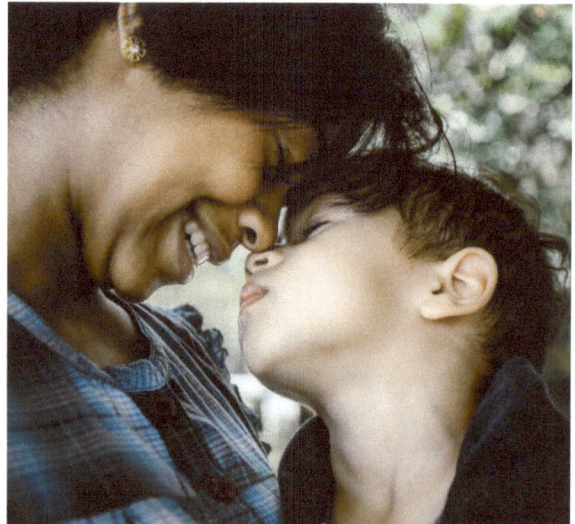
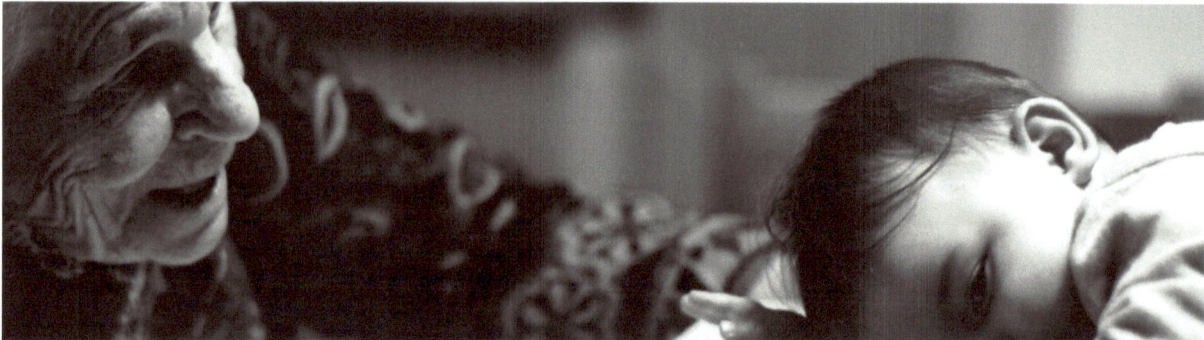

# CARE GIVING

Are you caring for children, the elderly, or someone faced with a health crisis? Perhaps you are taking care of your children and one of your parents as well. From the outside few can understand how exhausting it is to be a caregiver.

Caregivers need an extra dose of self-love and self-care. They have the least free room with which to step away and find time for themselves. There is no such thing as the end of the workday for someone taking care of children or other dependents. What is the solution?

## MINI WELLNESS BREAKS

Tiny wellness breaks can be spaced throughout the day of five to ten minutes; each can add up to a surge in your sense of well-being and contentment. Just a few minutes of meditation, reading, creating, learning, movement, time in nature, playing, or socializing can make all the difference. If you're exhausted and stretched thin mentally with worry, to-do lists, and work, then you won't know what to do when five minutes are available.

In a quiet moment write yourself a list of activities you would love to turn to for a moment of respite. Sign-up for that on-line Italian course, take out your sewing project, get out your tools and project plans, place your book on the counter. When five to ten minutes open up, you can turn directly to your chosen activity. Integrating children or elderly into the uplifting activities you enjoy is the best way to find time for events that will replenish you.

Just state what you would like to do for the next few minutes and ask that they do it with you. Afterward, tell them it's their turn to choose the future activity. You don't need to manipulate children or parents into participating. You have a right also to do events that bring you joy for a few minutes. If they refuse to join you, then accept their decision and engage in your activity anyway. Just a few minutes can refill your fuel tank and place you in a better place to give of yourself.

Create a schedule for movement. Yes, you probably are exhausted. So you don't feel like there is the energy in you to exercise. Just ten minutes three times a day add up to half an hour of moving your body and skyrocketing your health and well-being.

Write down a schedule for when you will do a few minutes of yoga, tai chi, dance, qi gong, or another form of movement. First thing in the morning, just before lunch, and late afternoon are optimal times to boost your energy levels without reaching for sugar or caffeine.

# Eating and drinking

## MINDFUL MEALS

Open up space and time to eat; make it an event. It doesn't matter if you are dining alone or in a decadent restaurant with beloved family or friends. Start treating each meal as an experience worthy of your full attention. Turn off the television, your phone, and set aside distractions. You may want to light a candle or take your meal outside to enjoy alfresco.

Take in the color of the food, the texture, the scent. Think of the farmers who grew the food and the travel of the food from the field to your plate.

Bless your food. You don't need to be religious or spiritual to be grateful. Changing how you eat your food will alter how your body digests and absorbs the nutrients and energy.

## EAT COLOR, EAT FRESH

Pay attention to the energy quality of the food you eat. Produce selected from a market of proud local farmers will nourish you. Plants sprayed with toxic chemicals, harvested by desperate and underpaid workers, and transported vast distances is not like the fresh produce picked from your garden. Avoid protein from mistreated, unhappy animals.

Opt for protein from happy animals allowed to range free outside. Above all don't become judgmental and obsessive about food. You don't need to allow guilt or shame to flood through you if you eat something you don't think is healthy. Instead, bless whatever food is in front of you with gratitude and ask that it nourish your body with vital health.

## SPICES

Depending on your inherent dosha constitution, spices can be a way to pack powerful antioxidants into your diet while giving your digestion system a detox.

Add ¼ of a teaspoon of turmeric spice, ½ teaspoon cinnamon, ¼ teaspoon ginger, ½ teaspoon black pepper, and ¼ teaspoon cardamom to a cup of almond milk, cashew, or coconut milk and warm. If you have a milk foaming machine, you can add everything to it and warm this way. You can drink this antioxidant and health packed latte first thing in the morning.

## Turmeric

Turmeric is arguably the healthiest spice. Turmeric contains curcumin, a potent healing compound. Researchers are fascinated with the power of turmeric; more than 5,000 clinical studies have been conducted to test turmeric's power in disease prevention and treatment. Turmeric has antioxidant, anti-inflammatory, and anti-cancer properties. Ongoing clinical trials are testing the power of the curcumin in turmeric to prevent and treat a wide variety of cancers and brain disease. Dr. Greger reveals in his scientifically researched book, *How Not to Die* that turmeric effectively fights against cancer-causing substances in clinical trials. A study in 2017 further supports the cancer-fighting potential of curcumin.

Curcumin was proven to be chemo preventative against a carcinogenic in a recent clinical trial. Even if you aren't concerned about cancer, adding some turmeric to your latte or oatmeal in the morning can act as a painkiller,

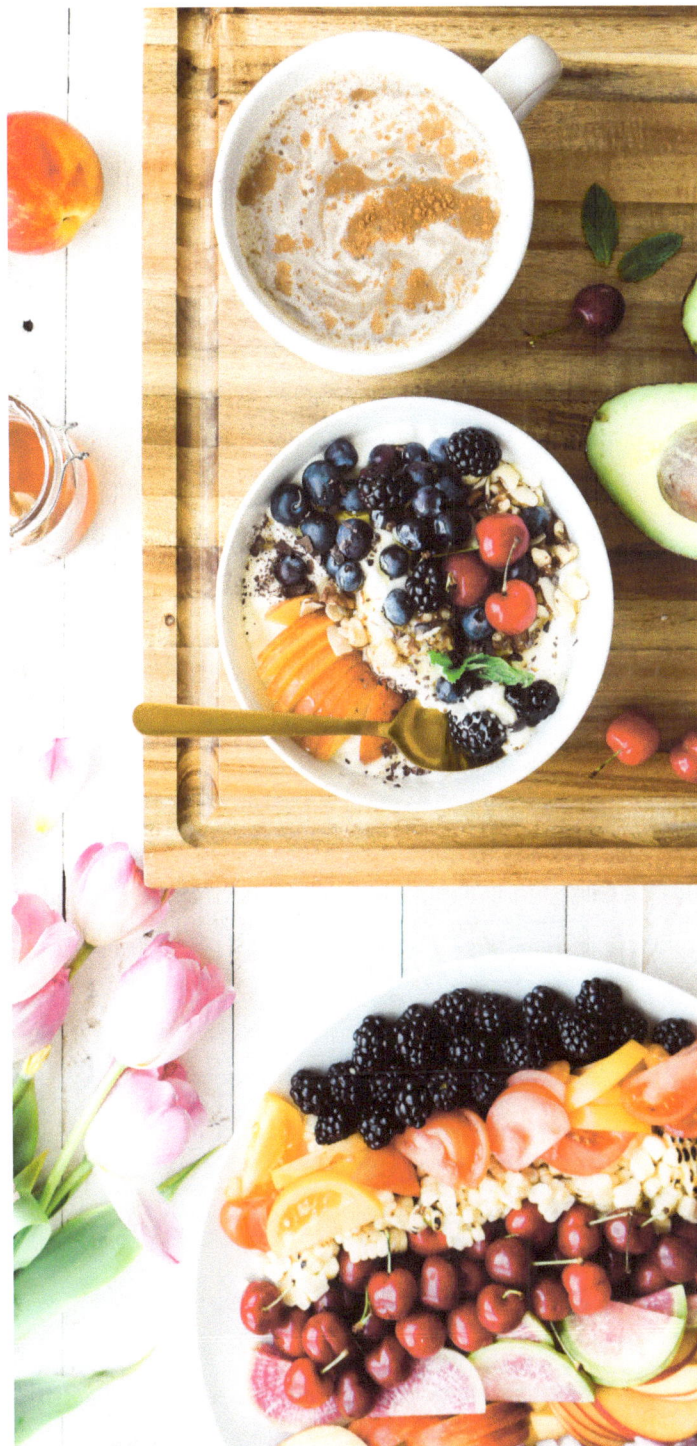

anti-inflammatory, antidepressant, and even improve your skin. With all the benefits of turmeric, you could add the rest of the spices to add flavor. Each spice in the latte contains significant health benefits as well.

## Cinnamon
Studies indicate that cinnamon could lower your blood sugar and has anti-inflammatory, antimicrobial, and antioxidant effects.

## Ginger
Ginger fights cancer, as well as being anti-inflammatory, anti-fungal and supports the digestive system, weight loss, and immunity. In a recent clinical study of ovarian cancer, researchers found ginger extract to have anticancer properties.

Ginger even worked the same or better when tested in clinical trials against leading pharmaceuticals to treat menstrual pain and migraines, without the adverse side effects of the expensive drugs. One hundred patients in a double-blinded randomized clinical trial were chosen at random to receive either the drug sumatriptan or ginger powder. The effectiveness of the treatment was recorded for the next five migraines.

What was the result? Are you guessing that the expensive drug's efficacy was higher than the low-cost ginger powder? The treatment of frequent migraine attacks with ginger powder was found in the clinical trial to be statistically comparable with the drug.

## Pepper
Stirring black pepper into your latte increases the potential efficacy of the curcumin by up to 2,000%! Besides being antibacterial and filled with antioxidants, the black pepper may also increase your body's resting metabolic rate, which can help you in weight control. Add a final dash of cardamom to your latte, and you could help prevent blood sugar spikes and reduce the ability of fat to develop around your middle.

## HEALTHY WEIGHT

You know diets don't work. It seems that every few months new diets come out as to which way of eating is the healthiest. Let's make it simple. Eat mostly plants. Aim to eat a rainbow of colors over the course of a week. Only eat freshly prepared foods and avoid processed foods. Add in spices to your diet such as ginger, cinnamon, cardamom, garlic, and others as well as herbs for flavor and health fortifying properties. Make sure you eat at least half a cup of raw veggies, like cut up red peppers, cucumbers, and carrots, before your main meal of the day. Fill at least half your plate with plants at dinner. Eat plenty of protein and healthy fats, such as high-quality olive oil, nuts, and avocados. Remember that grains, also whole grains, convert to sugar and eat them with moderation. Instead of always reaching for wheat, corn, or potatoes, aim to eat a variety of other options. Lentils, beans, and chickpeas are gluten-free, high in nutrition, and full of flavor. Spice up routine by making dishes such as sweet potatoes, bulgar wheat, quinoa, polenta, and couscous.

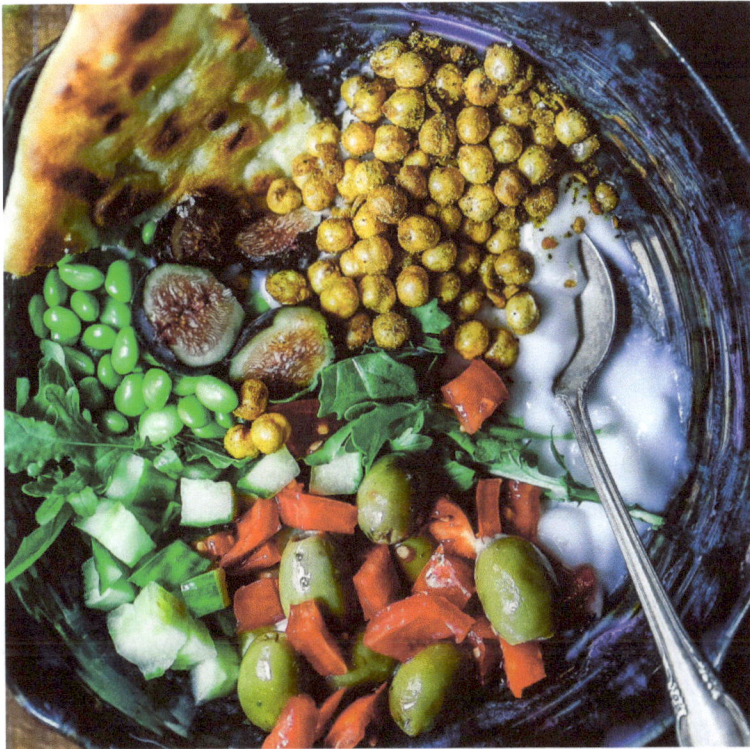

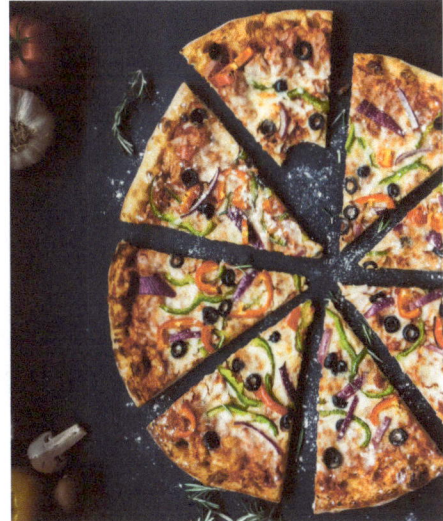

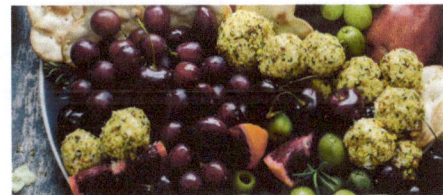

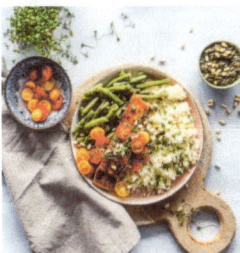

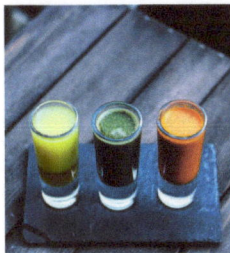

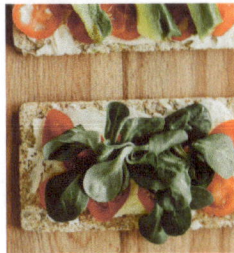

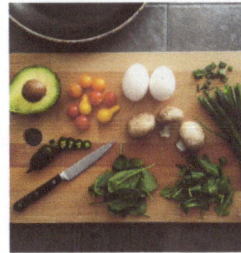

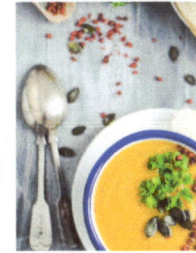

If you can't give up your daily dessert, like me, then bake it yourself from scratch. You will be able to reduce sugar and salt dramatically.

Do you need sugar with your coffee? See if you can substitute eating a square of 70% dark chocolate with raw or roasted almonds or walnuts instead.

## SNACKING & SAVORING

Always eat a treat with a raw veggie. For example, eat a carrot before that brownie. The high fiber of the carrot will fill you up and slow the rush of sugar from the brownie to your bloodstream. When you do eat a piece of cake, a bowl of chips, French fries, or anything else high in sugar, saturated fat, salt, or processed ingredients, then savor the food. Take your full attention to the present moment. Savor every bite. Release emotional ties to food. Relax and try to enjoy food again instead of controlling it, or letting it control you.

## FASTING

Once a week have a sugar free day where you only eat veggies, lentils, nuts, and healthy oils. A sugar vacation will allow your gut to detox, give your pancreas a break, and allow inflammation in your body to heal. It will also recalibrate your palate, so you are more sensitive to sweetness. A little bit of sweet will go much farther than before.

Once a week fast from eating anything until lunch time and drink only one black coffee, at least half a liter of pure water with freshly squeezed lemon, and unsweetened tea. The morning fast will give your digestion a break and allow your body to detox. Don't use your morning fast as an excuse to eat more calories or sugar the rest of the day.

## VITAMINS & MINERALS

Take a multivitamin which contains minerals imperative for health lacking in our diets, such as iodine, calcium, magnesium, and vitamin D. In the winter in the north you will need to up your vitamin D3 to 5,000 IU. Few women get enough magnesium, which can lead to osteoporosis as magnesium aids in the absorption of calcium. A lack of magnesium can also cause insomnia, lower quality of sleep, muscle aches, and itchy skin. Drink magnesium-rich mineral water or take an additional supplement to your multivitamin. Low iodine negatively impacts your health and the function of your thyroid and can cause hair loss. Iodine in salt is not enough. Be sure you are getting 12.5 mg per day.

## DIGESTION WALK

Walking thirty minutes a day not only increases your resilience to stress and burnout; it is also a magic remedy for the digestive system. You don't need to walk thirty minutes at once to get all the benefits. Make it a ritual to go for a five to fifteen-minute walk every day after lunch and again after dinner to aide your body in the digestion process. Use the walk as an opportunity to search for beauty and flow into the present moment.

If your thoughts don't come to stillness, you can repeat a mantra internally, such as Ananda Hum, which means, I am pure bliss or Hum Sa, I am that.

Alternatively, you can bring your attention to the sounds around you, the feel of your clothes against your skin, the smell of the flowers, the sensation of placing one foot in front of the other, and the rise and fall of your breathing.

## PURE WATER & TEAS

Opt for pure water and unsweetened teas. Smoothies and fruit juices seem healthy but are packed with sugar. Eating the whole fruit is healthy, but juice is not. You need the fiber in the entire fruit, which slows the release of the sugar to your bloodstream.

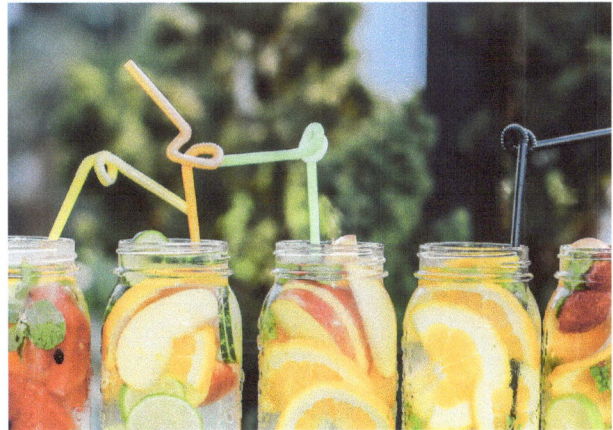

## FOOD ENERGY TESTING

You can test whether a food type is positive or negative for your body, according to Donna Eden. Take the food in your hand and press it to your solar plexuses. Your body needs the food type if the food pulls you forward. Your body doesn't want the energy of the food if you lean backward. The food is neutral for you if you remain standing straight up.

# YOGA FOR DIGESTION

**1**

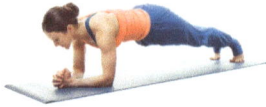

## Forearm Plank

-Hold plank pose for 10 deep, slow breaths.
-Engage your abs.
-Lengthen your tailbone towards your heels.

**2**

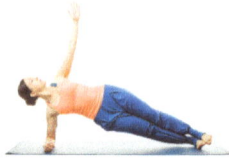

## Side Plank

-Roll over onto your forearm. Stack your feet. Lift your hips away from the floor.
-Lift he pelvic floor. Pull the navel in.
-Repeat on other side.

**3**

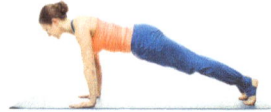

## Plank

-Bring shoulders over wrists. Lift the pelvic floor. Engage abs.
-Lengthen your low back. Broaden across the shoulders.
-Gaze soft.

**4**

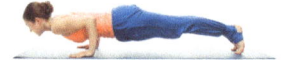

## Chaturanga

-Shift forward on your toes. Stack shoulders over wrists.
-Squeeze elbows in to the ribcage as you lower down in one line.
-Keep shoulders back.

**5**

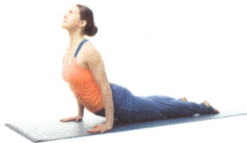

## Urdhva Mukha

-Lift the heart forward and through the arms.
-Press into the tops of the feet. Lift the legs.
-Roll shoulders back and down the spine.
-Micro-bend the arms.

**6**

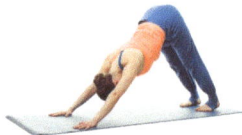

## Adho Mukha

-Spread fingers wide.
-Press the hips back as you push out of the arms.
-Lengthen the spine.
-Melt the heels down.
-Pull the belly inwards.

**7**

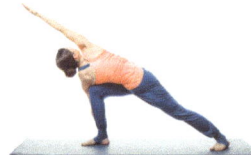

## Parivrtta Parsvakonasana

-Bring your left elbow to the outside of your right knee. Lengthen.
-Twist. Revolve the heart up to the sky.
-Squeeze hips in.

**8**

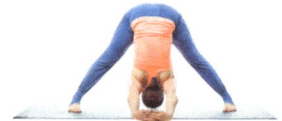

## Prasarita Padottanasana

-Grab your big toes.
-Fold forward in between your legs.
-Engage the legs.
-Lengthen the spine.
-Use the abs to fold.

Hold each pose for ten deep, slow, even breaths with sound in and out the nose, creating a wave like sound with your breathing by constricting the back of the throat. Repeat the flow on the opposite side and then relax in Shavasana for 5-10 minutes.

**9**

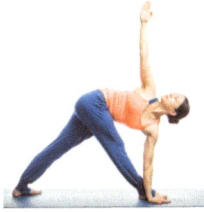

### Parivrtta Trikonasana

-Bring your right foot forward. Square the hips to the front.
-Bring your left hand outside the right foot.
-Lengthen, then twist.

**10**

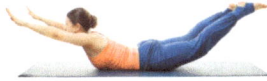

### Salabhasana

-Press the hips into the mat. Lift your arms and legs up. Lengthen and lift higher.
-Squeeze inner thighs into mid line.
-Shoulders on back.

**11**

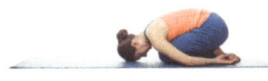

### Balasana

-Bring your feet together, open your knees, hips to heels, melt your forehead to the floor.
-Allow the back body to soften. Breathe.

**12**

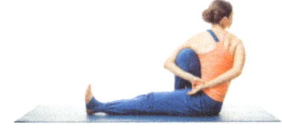

### Matsyendrasana

-Bend your right leg.
-Ground both sitting bones down.
-Bring your left elbow to the outside of the right knee or around the knee. Twist.

**13**

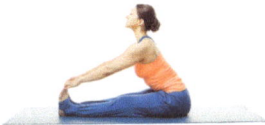

### Paschimottanasana

-Straighten both legs.
-Tilt pelvis forward.
-Press hamstrings into the mat. Long spine.
-Lift the pelvic floor; use the belly to pull you forward.

**14**

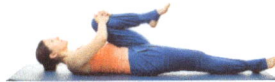

### Knee to Chest

-Grab your left knee and pull it into your chest.
-Press the low back into the floor.
-Relax your shoulders away from your ears.

**15**

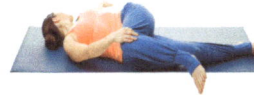

### Supta Matsyendrasana

-Lift the hips. Shift hips to right.
-Bend left knee and take it across the body.
-Stretch arms out.
-Look at left hand.

**16**

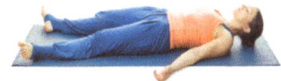

### Shavasana

-Straighten both legs.
-Roll onto your back. You can place a bolster under your knees.
-Pull the shoulder blades on your back.
-Relax everything.

# BUDDHA VEGGIE BOWL

## VEGETABLES

2 Tablespoon olive, melted coconut, or avocado oil

2 small sweets potatoes (halved) and 1 small/medium butternut squash, peeled, seeded, and cubed

¼ teaspoon each salt + pepper

Shredded cabbage and carrots, fresh spinach, and half an avocado per serving

## CHICKPEAS

1 15-ounce chickpeas (drained, rinsed + patted dry)

1 teaspoon cumin

¾ teaspoon chili powder

¾ teaspoon garlic powder

¼ teaspoon each salt + pepper

½ teaspoon oregano (optional)

¼ teaspoon turmeric (optional)

## TAHINI SAUCE (OPTIONAL)

¼ cup tahini

1 Tablespoon maple syrup

½ medium lemon (juiced)

2-4 Tablespoon hot water (to thin)

## Instructions

Preheat oven to 200 degrees Celsius and line a baking sheet with parchment paper. Peel, de-seed, and cube the squash and halve the sweet potatoes and toss with one to two tablespoons of olive oil, salt, pepper, and cumin seeds.

Place the sweet potatoes and squash on a bare baking sheet. Roast in the over for 10 minutes – 20 minutes, or until soft but not mushy.

While vegetables are roasting, heat one tablespoon of olive oil on the stove. Add your drained chickpeas to the pan with the 3/4 teaspoon chili powder, 3/4 teaspoon garlic powder, 1 teaspoon cumin and 1/4 teaspoon each salt and pepper. Stir over medium heat for about ten minutes, or until the chickpeas are brown.

Mix the tahini, lemon juice, and maple syrup together for the sauce and then add the two to four tablespoons of hot water. To serve: Add the half of avocado, spinach leaves, shredded red cabbage and carrots to each bowl along with the roasted sweet potatoes, squash, and sautéed chickpeas. Drizzle with the Tahini sauce.

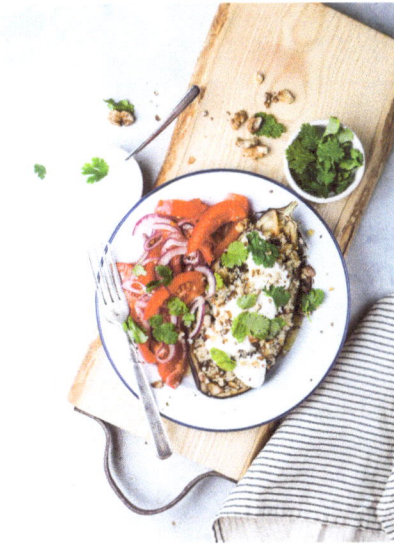
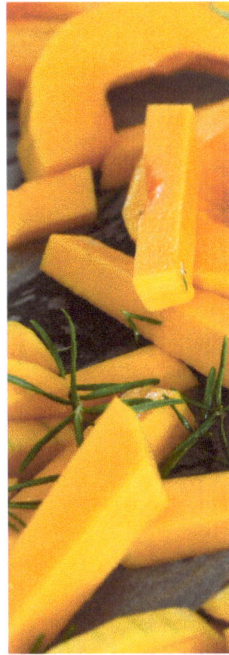
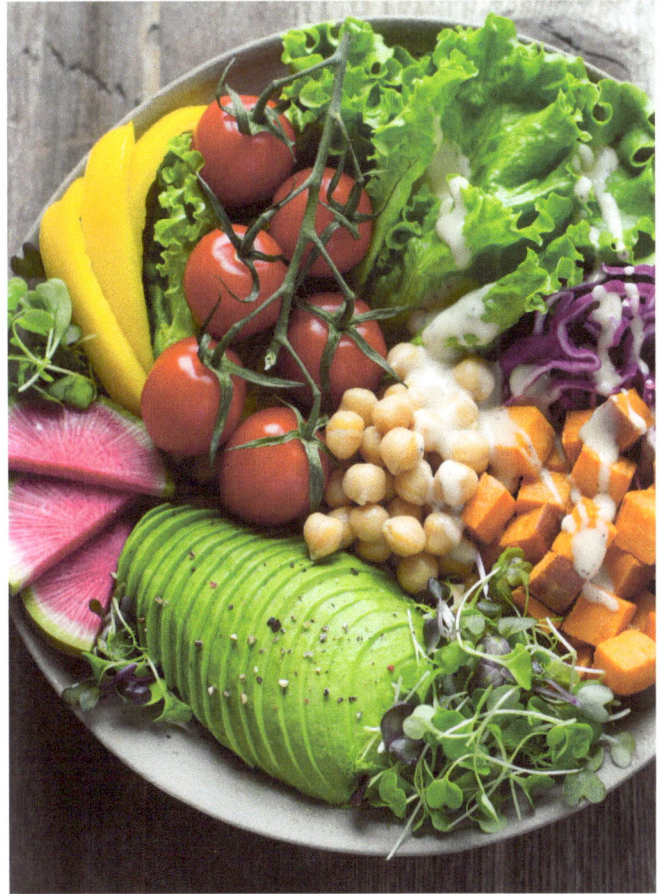
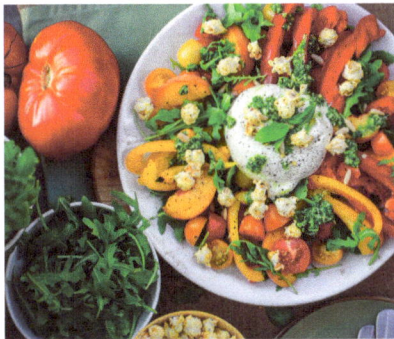
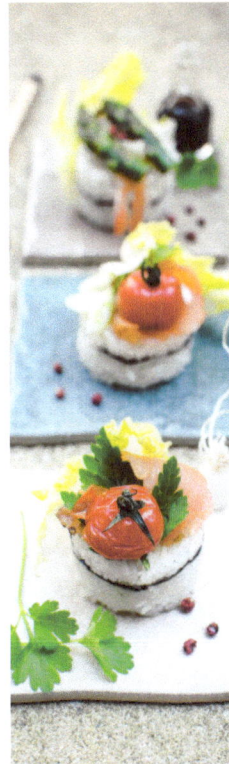
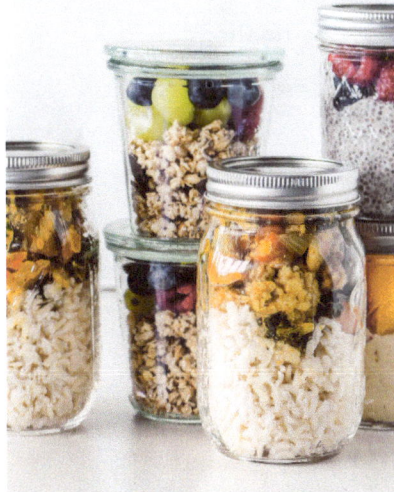
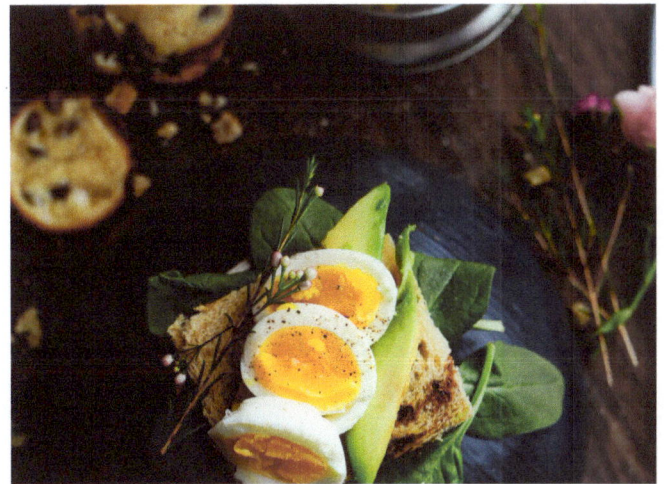

It's all in the sauce. Make up a quick sauce to add to your combination of grain, vegetables, and protein to add flavor, nutrients and variety. All of these green sauces are packed with nourishing, healthy goodness and delicious on veggie wraps, Buddha bowls, salads, over pasta, or on wholegrain toast, beans, chickpeas, lentils, rice, hummus, roasted vegetables, quinoa, or couscous.

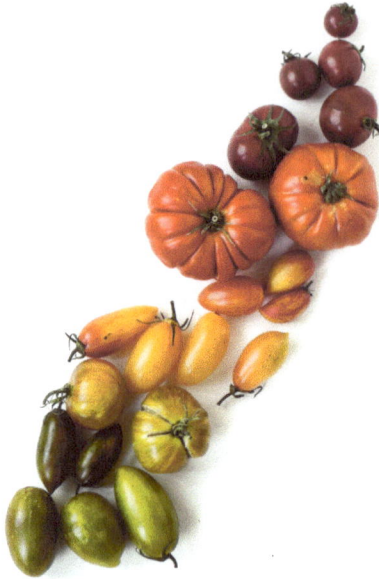

## Chimichurri

¼ cup coarsely chopped parsley
3 tablespoons red wine vinegar
4 large garlic cloves
Minced 2 tablespoons oregano leaves
2 teaspoons crushed red pepper
Salt and freshly ground pepper to taste

½ cup extra-virgin olive oil

Put the parsley, vinegar, garlic, oregano and crushed red pepper into a food processor and mix until smooth. Place into a serving dish and then pour the olive oil over the mixture. Refrigerate for at least 20 minutes.

## Chermoula

2  large bunches of cilantro leaves
1 large bunch of parsley leaves
3 to 4  garlic cloves halved, green shoots removed
½ to ¾  teaspoon salt (optional)
2  teaspoons ground cumin seed
1  teaspoon sweet paprika
½  teaspoon ground coriander seeds
⅛  teaspoon cayenne
⅓ to ½  cup extra virgin olive oil

¼ cup freshly squeezed lemon juice

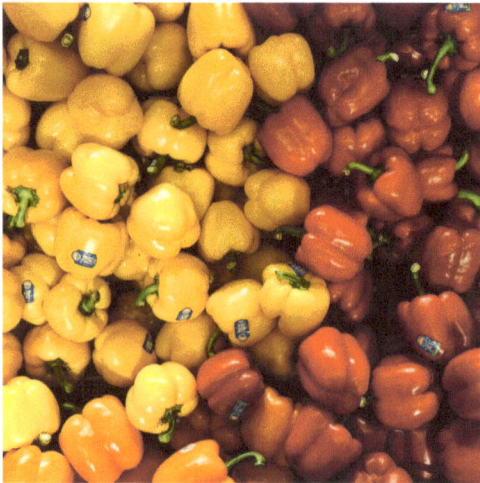

Add cilantro, parsley garlic cloves, cumin, coriander seeds, cayenne and salt into a food processor and process. Add the olive oil and lemon juice and puree.

108

## Salsa Verde

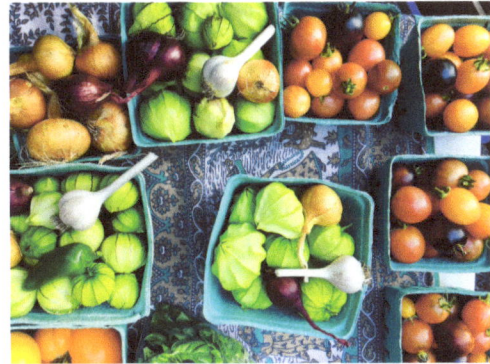

About 12 medium tomatillos husked and rinsed
1 jalapeños (Optional. Omit if you are a PITTA
½ a medium sized onion
1 Bunch of fresh cilantro leaves or more to taste
1-2 tablespoons medium limes, juiced
½ to 1 teaspoon salt, to taste

Optional variation: 1 avocado, for creamy salsa

Preheat your oven to 200 Celsius and place the tomatillos and jalapeño on a baking sheet and broil until they're blackened in spots, about 5 minutes and then flip. Tomatillos look like green tomatoes covered in a husk. Add the cilantro, lime juice, salt and onion and garlic to your food processor and blend.

Next, add the tomatillos and peppers to the processor and blend until smooth. You can also let the salsa cool and then add an avocado for a creamier sauce.

## Pesto

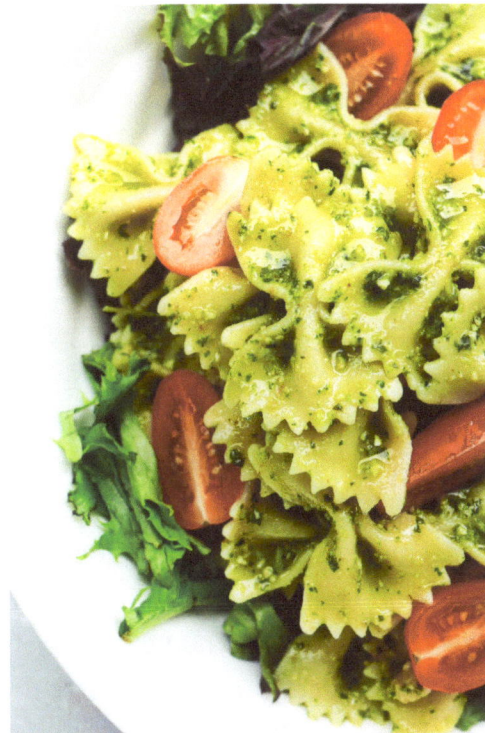

 2 cups fresh basil leaves, packed (can sub half the basil leaves with baby spinach)
½ cup freshly grated Romano or Parmesan - Reggiano cheese (about 2 ounces)
½ cup extra virgin olive oil
⅓ cup pine nuts (can sub chopped walnuts)
3 garlic cloves, minced (about 3 teaspoons)
¼ teaspoon salt, more to taste

a dash of freshly ground black pepper

Add the pine nuts and the basil to your food processor first and blend before adding the garlic and the cheese. Pulse a few times before adding the olive oil in a slow stream into the food processor while it blends to help it emulsify.

## Chile-Herb Dipping Sauce

1 tablespoon jasmine or other long-grain rice
6 to 8 dried whole Thai chilies
1 heaping tablespoon finely chopped scallion
2 tablespoons finely chopped fresh mint
2 tablespoons finely chopped fresh cilantro
2 teaspoons sugar
3 tablespoons Thai or Vietnamese fish sauce

⅓ cup fresh lime juice

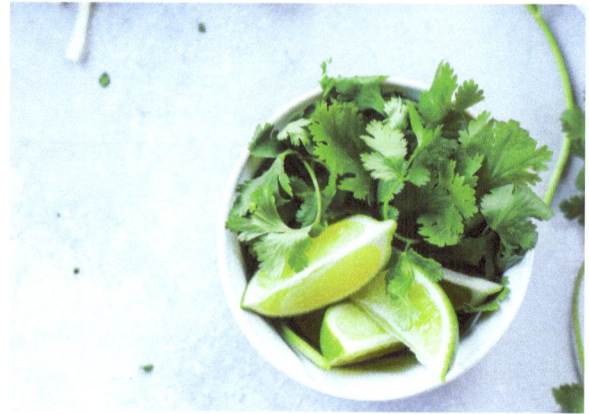

Add the rice to a pan and cook over medium heat until the rice is lightly toasted, about one minute and then place the rice to cool in a bowl.

Add the chilies to the pan and cook over medium heat for one minute and then set aside to cool. Add the rice to your food processor and blend until you have a powder and then return to the bowl. Add the chilies to the food processor and blend.

Mix the chilies into the bowl together the powdered rice, scallion, cilantro, sugar, fish sauce, mint, and lime juice.

## Zhoug

4 medium cloves garlic
2 bunches fresh cilantro leaves
2 medium jalapeños without seeds
1 teaspoon fine sea salt
1 teaspoon ground cardamom
½ teaspoon sesame seeds
½ teaspoon ground cumin
¼ teaspoon red pepper flakes
¾ cup extra-virgin olive oil

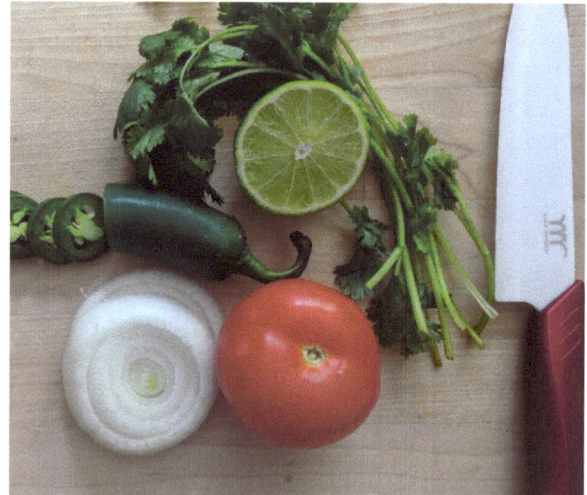

Pulse the garlic in your food processor until roughly chopped and then add the cilantro, jalapeño, red pepper, cumin, salt, and cardamom and blend until fine. Next, add the olive oil into the food processor as it continue to blend. Cover and place in the fridge for at least an hour before serving.

## Green Chutney

1 cup chopped coriander leaves
¼ inch fresh ginger
1 teaspoon groundnuts
½ teaspoon cumin seeds
2 teaspoons fresh coconut
2 garlic cloves
1 green chili without seeds
1 teaspoon lemon juice
½ teaspoon sugar; ½ teaspoon salt
1 tablespoon water

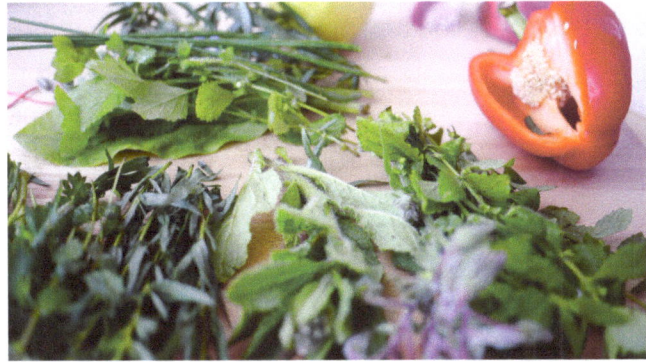

Blend the coconut, sesame seeds, cumin seeds, and groundnuts in your food processor until powdery and then add the garlic chili, ginger, sugar, salt, lemon juice, water and coriander leaves. Mix until smooth, adding water or lemon juice to taste.

## Maslala Sauce

5 cloves garlic
2 tablespoons crushed fresh ginger
3 tablespoon garam masala
1 tablespoon chili powder
1 tablespoon turmeric
1 tablespoon cumin
1 ¼ teaspoons ground cloves
2 teaspoons salt
¼ teaspoon cayenne pepper
2 onions and a small pile of cilantro stems
1 cup almonds

Juice of one lemon
1 ½ cups tomato puree + ½ cup water

1 14-ounce coconut milk

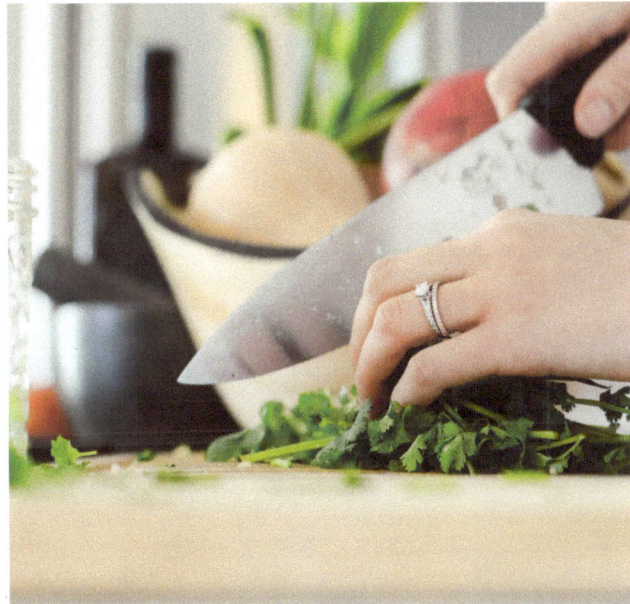

Place the garlic, fresh ginger, garam Masala, chili powder, turmeric, cumin, ground cloves, salt, cayenne pepper, cilantro stems, onions, almonds, and lemon into your food processor and blend. Place in a jar. Heat olive oil in a pan and add ¼ cup of your masala paste from the jar to your pan and place the rest of your masala paste into the fridge. Stir the masala paste in the pan for five minutes and then add the water and tomato puree. Let simmer on low heat for ten minutes before adding the coconut milk. Simmer ten minutes more minutes and it is ready to serve.

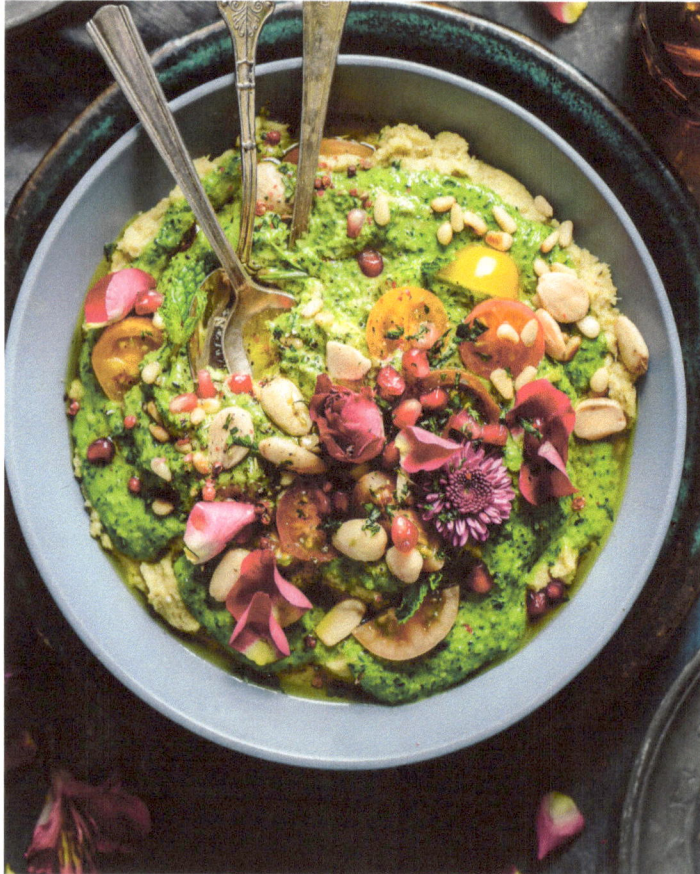

## Green Magic Sauce

1 avocado
1 cup packed parsley and cilantro leaves (combined)
1 jalapeño, ribs and seeds removed
2 cloves garlic
Juice of one lime (or two – get lots of lime goodness in there!)
½ cup water
½ cup olive oil
1 teaspoon salt
½ cup pistachios (optional)

Mix the avocado, parsley, cilantro, jalapeño, garlic cloves, lime, water, and salt in the food processor and then slowly add in the olive oil. Add the optional pistachios last and blend until you get your desired smoothness.

# BUDDHA OATMEAL BOWL INGREDIENTS

1 cup rolled, old fashion oats for every one cup milk, water, or yogurt you add
1 tablespoon chia seeds
½ teaspoon cinnamon
¼ teaspoon ginger
¼ teaspoon cardamom

¼ teaspoon nutmeg

## Topping options:

Sliced strawberries, raspberries, or bananas
Pomegranate seeds and blueberries
Cherries and grated vanilla bean

Sautéed bananas or apples with cinnamon

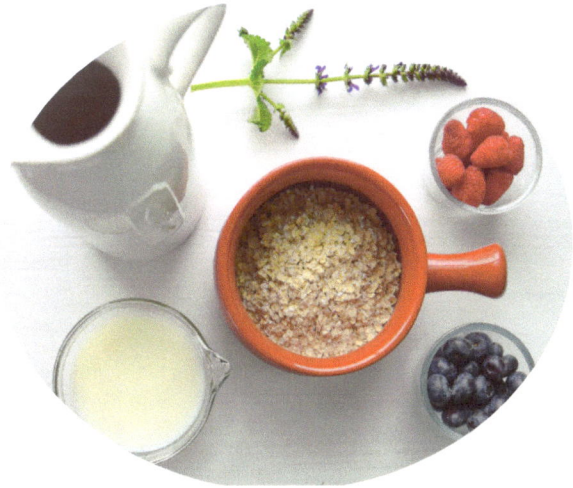

Roast almond silvers, cashews, walnuts, or pecans in a skillet until golden brown, cool, and store in a jar for the week. Add into of your Buddha oatmeal bowl after cooking or once taken out of the refrigerator.

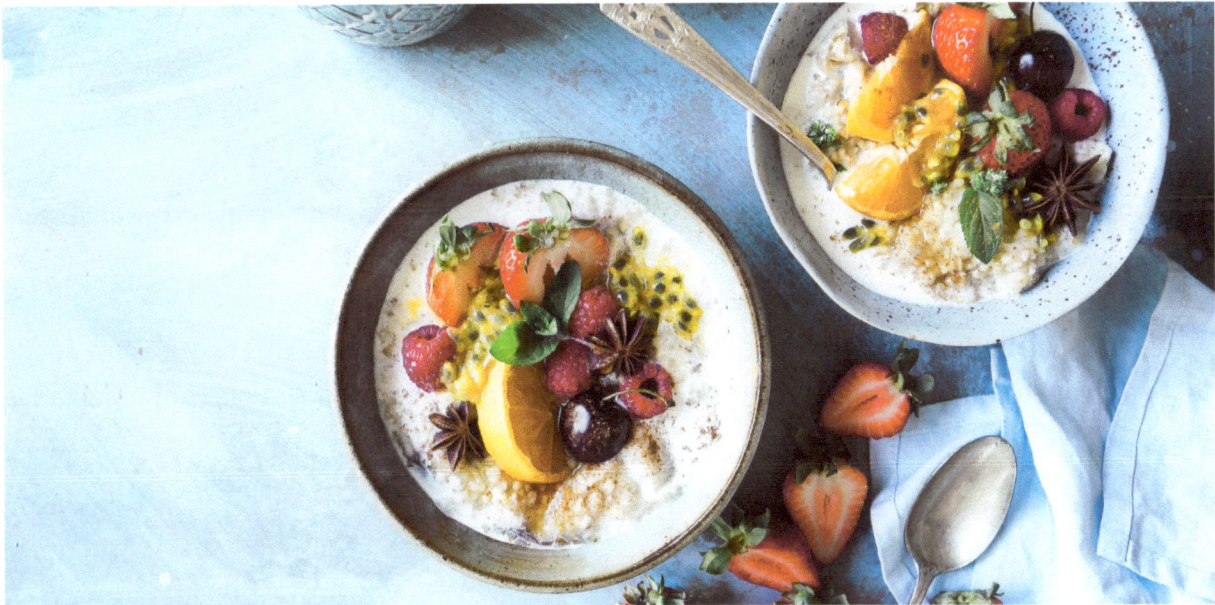

## OVERNIGHT BUDDHA OATMEAL JARS

Add one cup of old fashioned oats to one cup milk, yogurt, or water and place in a glass jar with the spices and chia seeds. Add fresh cut fruit selection on top and store in the fridge overnight. Add your nuts on top in the morning.

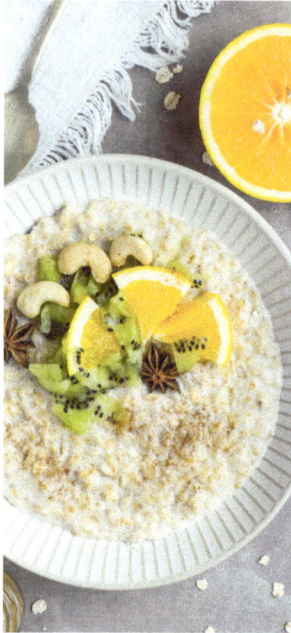

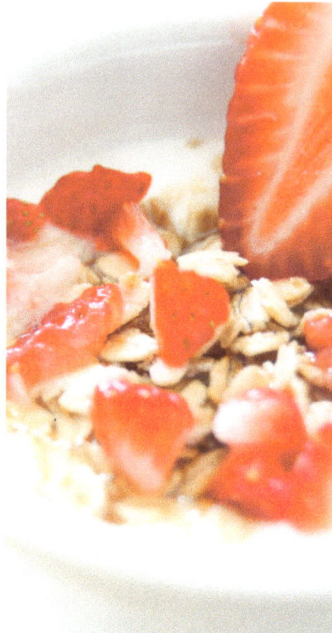

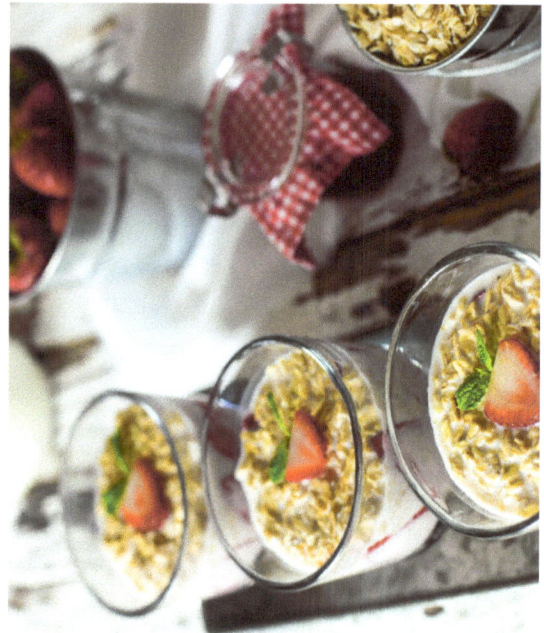

## HOT BUDDHA OATMEAL BOWL

Add one cup of old fashioned oats to every cup of milk or water you need and add your spices. Bring to a boil, then reduce heat to low. Next simmer uncovered for 3 to 5 minutes until thickened, stirring occasionally. Remove from heat and let cool slightly.

   Last add blueberries, strawberries or your selection of fruit and nuts as well as your chia seeds to your oatmeal; add honey or maple syrup to sweeten as desired. Enjoy a glass of organic tea to rehydrate.

# Eat Mood Enhancing Foods

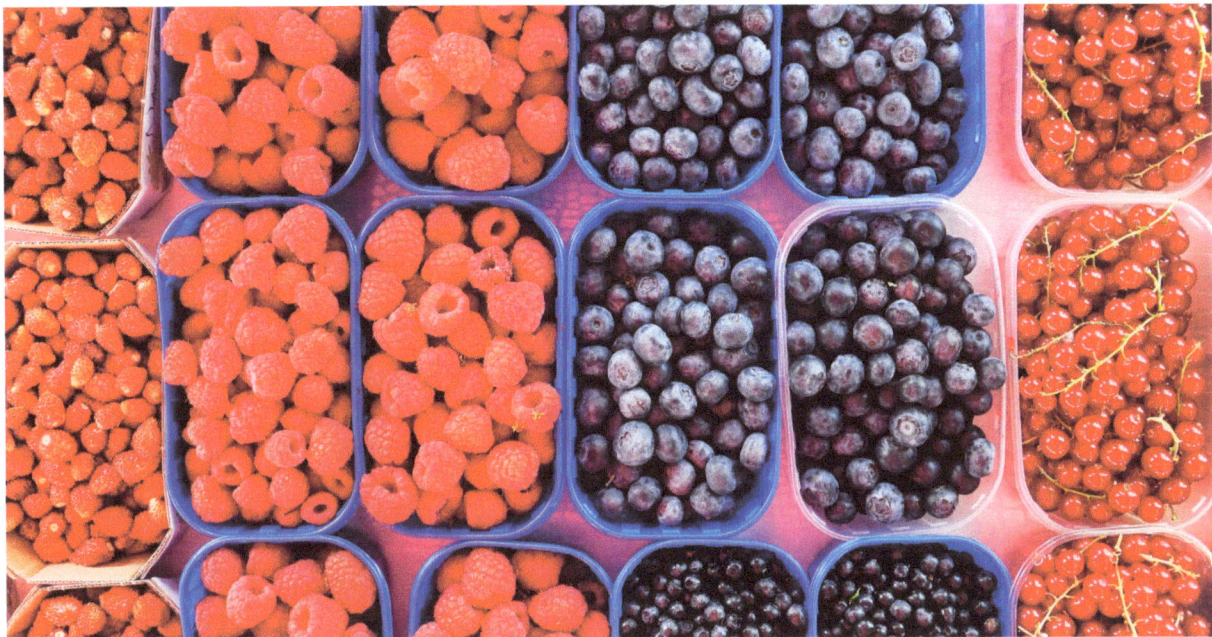

You know that eating a whole food diet comprised of vegetables, fruits, whole grains, proteins, and lots of pure water will increase your health, vitality, and happiness. You also know that processed foods and sugar cause inflammation and increase your risk of a long list of chronic diseases. The trouble is when you are standing in front of an ice-cream stand, or a birthday cake, or a pile of French fries. There is nothing wrong with you if you can't stop yourself from eating those sugar-filled and fatty foods. Stress, bacterial, parasitic invasions, and trauma can force your hand to reach out for unhealthy foods. Reach for healthy endorphin boosting foods as a go-to replacement for unhealthy choices.

Endomorphism-stimulating foods boast high levels of the vitamins and minerals that work in boosting your mood, like vitamin B12, vitamin C, zinc, potassium, and iron. The foods on the following pages will naturally lift your mood without the high dose of sugar, salt, or fat.

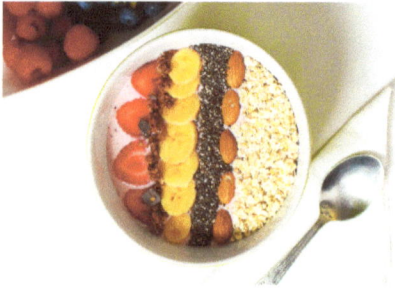

**Chia Seeds & Flax Seeds**
High in omega-3 fatty acids, a teaspoon of chia and flax seeds is high in vitamins and minerals and highly beneficial for not only the production of endorphins, but also your digestive, heart, bone health, and energy levels.

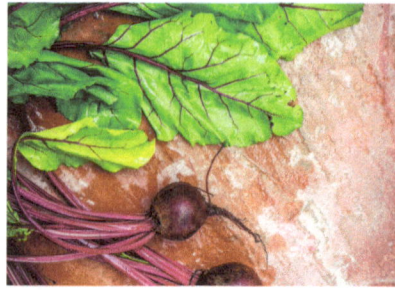

**Beetroot**
One of the top ten vegetables highest in antioxidants, beetroot will boost your production of immune-boosting white blood cells and is the juice athletes drink for more stamina. The betaine in beetroot triggers dopamine.

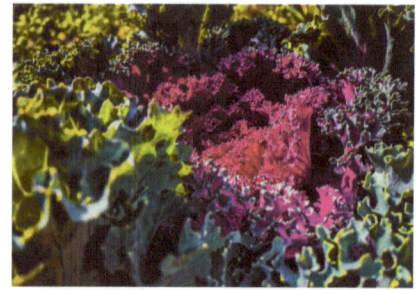

**Kale, Spinach, Rocket, Broccoli**
B Vitamins are essential for the production of serotonin, but stress depletes our bodies of this essential vitamin. Increase your consumption of leafy greens to support the production of serotonin, and dopamine in your body.

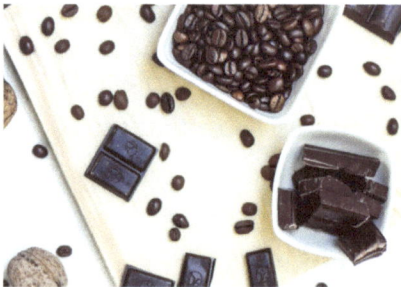

**Vanilla Bean**
Vanilla bean can increase the functioning of your neurotransmitters, reduce anxiety, and is high in B vitamins.

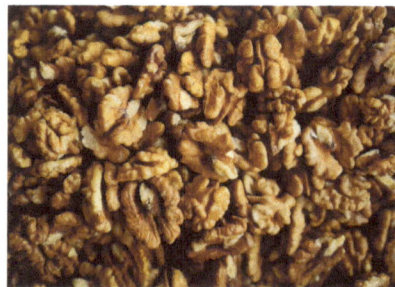

**Walnuts**
Walnuts are rich in omega-6 and omega-3 fatty acids and contains minerals like magnesium, iron, and potassium.

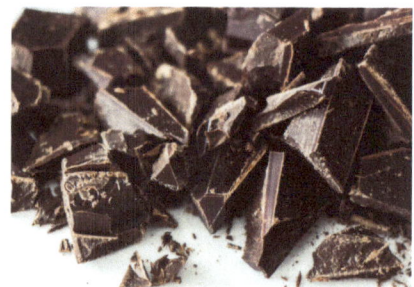

**70% Dark Chocolate**
Cacao stimulates the release of endorphins and the neurotransmitter serotonin. It is high in polyphenols and antioxidants.

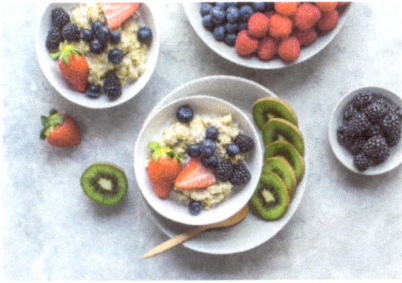

**Breakfast**

Add 1 teaspoon of chia and flaxseeds (ground) to your oatmeal, or muesli. Eat natural yogurt with berries, which is full of probiotics which assist in improving mood and your immune system.

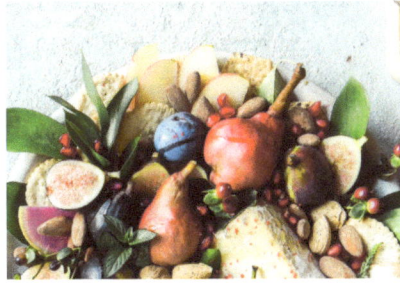

**Snack**

Eating two to five walnuts, cashews, or almonds with a small piece of dark chocolate will satisfy your need for a treat and boost your mood and energy.

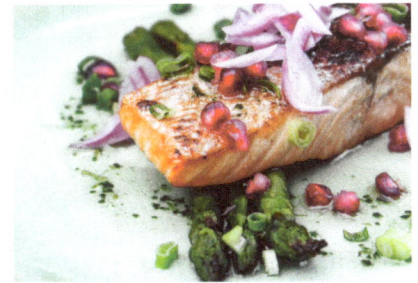

**Lunch or Dinner**

Add kale, Swiss chard, spinach, avocado, and beetroot to your salad. Eat wild salmon, which is high in omega-3 fatty acids and add a whole grain for energy.

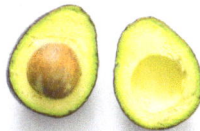

**Avocados**

Avocados have choline, which facilitates higher dopamine and serotonin levels. High in healthy fat, they add glow to hair and skin.

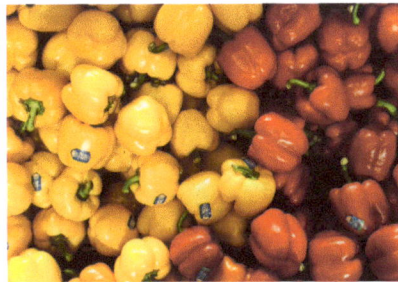

**Peppers**

Chili peppers have exceptionally high levels of capsaicin, a substance that triggers endorphin release. Spice up veggies.

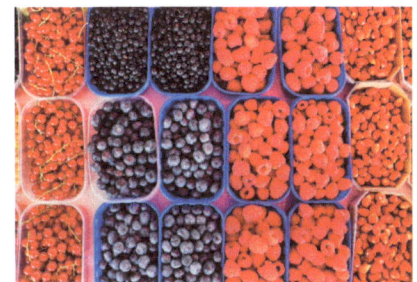

**Berries**

Berries such as blueberries have anthocyanidins and anthocyanins which help lift your mood.

# Relaxing after work

## WORK TO HOME TRANSITION

What is the first thing you do when you get home from work, or transition out of your workday? Do you rush right from your workday into your evening chores as soon as you get home? Do you slump onto a sofa when you get home and find it difficult to get up again? Do you reach for a glass of wine or entertainment?

Most people struggle to unclench from work and unfurl into relaxation. Wired but tired after a long work day, most people aren't in a state of being conducive to play, create, exercise, social-ize, or engage in hobbies that feed their joy.

Part of the solution is changing the structure and approach to the workday itself. Infusing the work day with wellness can cause you to end the day with energy to relish your free time. Set yourself up to end the workday with satisfaction and well-being:

-Set a clear intention for high-energy early morning work hours and apply goal-directed productivity.

-Introduce quality work breaks.

-Listen to your body and leverage breath-work, acupressure, and self-massage to release stress and tension throughout the day, so it doesn't build up.

-Consume wellness-enhancing food and drink.

-Optimize your work atmosphere to spark joy.

## BREATH WORK

Create a ritual when you first get home to shed any clinging tension, stress, or anxiety and rest your body. Place your belongings in their 'homes', wash your hands, perhaps change into more comfortable free-time clothing, and then lay down flat on your back on the floor for five to ten minutes. Do not lay on a bed, nor a sofa or chair. Laying flat on the floor is not something most

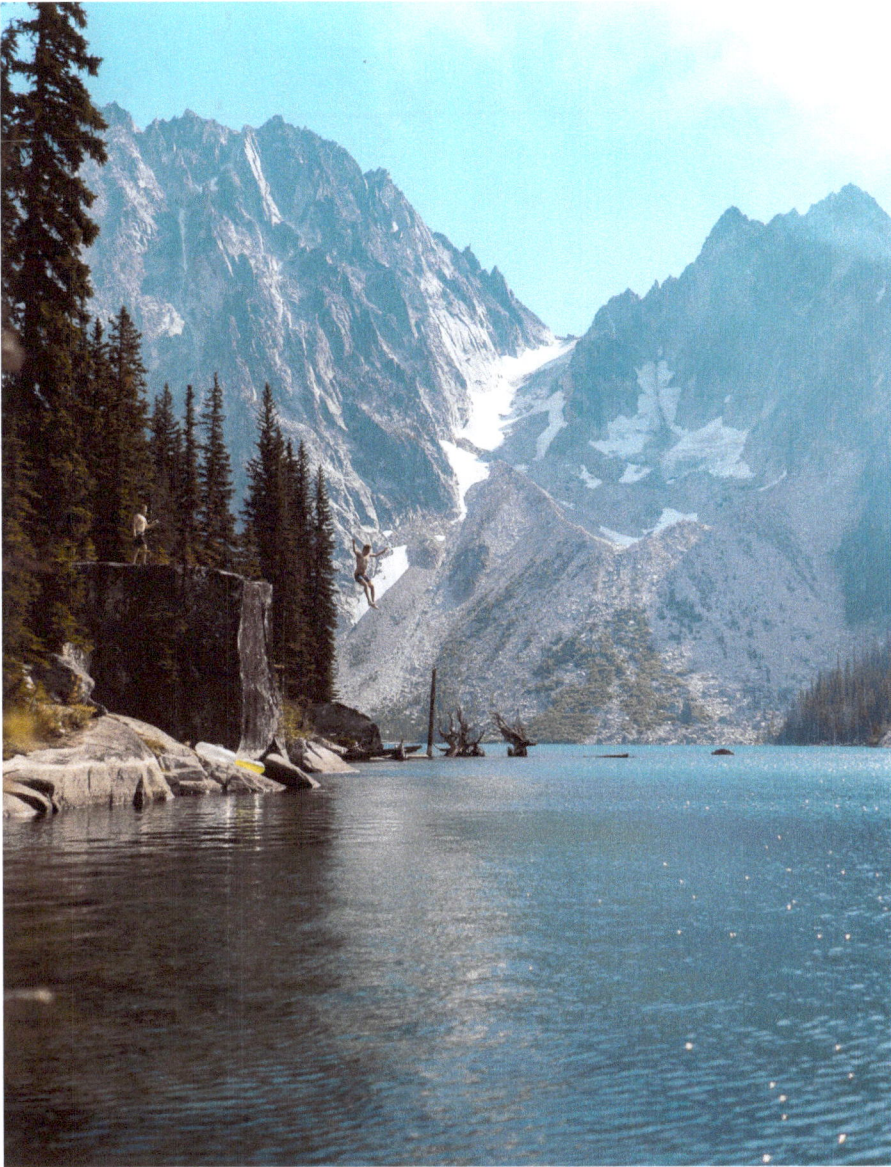
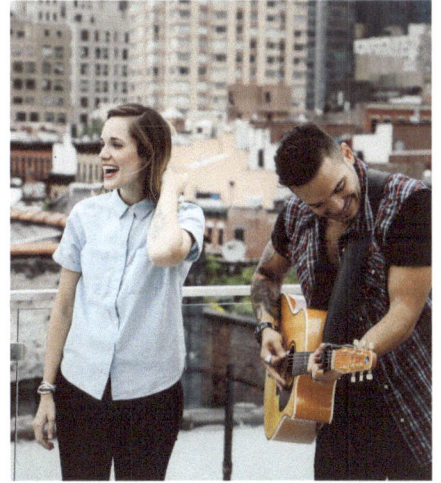
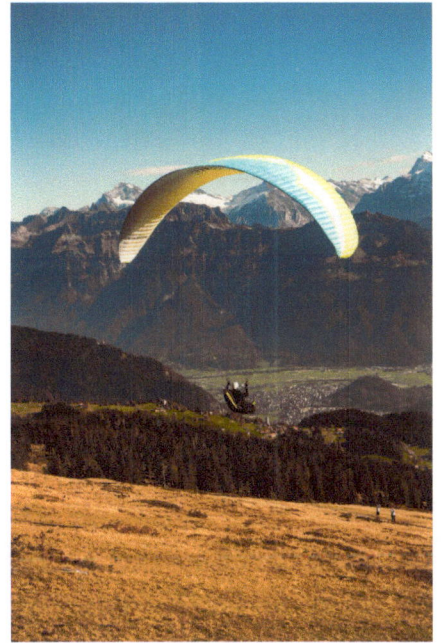
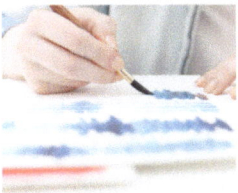
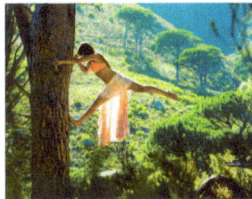
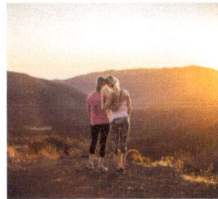
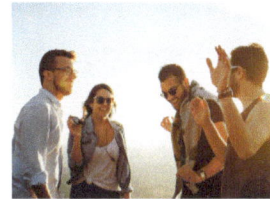
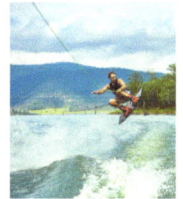

adults regularly do. Stretch your legs out long. Rest your arms by your sides. Allow your body to grow heavy, relax your shoulders down your back, and open your palms to the ceiling. Breathe in through your nose to the count of four. Breathe out through your mouth to the count of eight. Repeat five times and then let your body breathe you.

Roll over on to your right side at the end of five to ten minutes and press into your palms to rise to sit. Pause for a breath before you stand up. Allowing your body to rest in savasana as soon as you get home will activate your parasympathetic nervous system and shift you out of the stress state. If you aren't stressed, but exhausted, then a few minutes in savasana will recharge your batteries for your free hours. You may be hesitant to lay down when you first get home.

Chores, children, and dinner to make can make it seem indulgent to take ten minutes to rest and replenish. Or you may feel so fatigued that you fear laying down will mean you won't be able to summon the will power to accomplish your evening chores. Let the fear go. Taking a few minutes in savasana will begin to work its magic in as little as one week. You will be re-wiring your body and mind to shift out of action, into deep relaxation and replenishment, and back into action. Your energy, willpower, sense of inner balance, and contentment will get a boost.

## TIMELESSNESS + DIGITAL DETOX

Melting away from time is one of the best ways to escape the snake squeezing coils of stress. It's easy to lose track of time while surfing the Internet, on social media, or binging watching television. Falling into the quicksand of the digital will not move you forward on your journey to vitality, inner balance, and joy.

Set aside thirty to sixty minutes in the evening to disconnect from all things digital, set a timer, and release from time. Meditation is the best way to enter a state of timelessness.

You began your day with a few minutes of meditation, which will make it easier to release your monkey mind from seizing your attention. Commit to a 21 Day Meditation challenge to witness how an inner spaciousness opens up a place for more abundance, health, and happiness to flow into your life. Silence can be profoundly healing and stress-relieving. Open up space and time to soak up silence. Reading a book can allow your body to achieve a state of relaxation of higher rejuvenating quality than watching television. The mind is stimulated and activated more inter-actively while the body rests. Unlike while watching TV, you will fall asleep if you are exhausted, allowing you to slip into restorative sleep if you are deprived. Creating is an ideal way to slip into the timeless. You can return to the project you worked on for a few minutes in the morning. Feel too tired to write, color, knit, paint, craft, sculpt, or cook up a new recipe? Try setting a timer for twenty minutes and working on your project for just a few minutes.

Only a small dose of creating can sweep you up into an uplifted state of being. Learning something interesting just for its fascination can allow time and space to fall away.

Movement is a gorgeous way to use your digital detox time. You may love the intensity of a high-octane spinning or power yoga class. Gentle forms of exercise such as yin yoga, tai chi, and qi gong improve fitness, suppleness, mind-body awareness, and instill a current of calm. Dance is also a magical way to ignite joy. Terrible at dancing? Who cares? If you would like to improve though, take a class. You're never too old to learn. Is a dance class too intimidating? Close the curtains and learn from a course online.

Nature awaken wonder and a sense of connection to all things. Scientific studies found that participants who gardened were not only happier but healthier than the control group. Walking in a forest has been shown through scientific studies to lower stress hormones in the body and even boost the immune system. You can turn your walk into a moving meditation by keeping your focus on the present instead of ruminating in the past or the future. Repeating a mantra mentally, such as Hum Sa, OM, or Om Namah Shivaya, can keep your thoughts from dragging you away from the present like wild horses. If your mind strays from the mantra, merely label the distraction, like 'planning', and return to the mantra.

Playing isn't something most adults do regularly anymore. Being silly, laughing, and doing something without attachment to a goal or result reawakens the fun side of our personalities. Let care and tension slip away. Pull out some board games, go out and build a snowman, take a trip down a hill on a sled, frolic in the waves, build a sandcastle, play hide and seek. Take the clock backward and rekindle the childlike innocence and fun in you.

Socializing with family or friends can be a heartwarming and fortifying way to invest your free time after work. Scheduling quality time with family, friends, and making time for new connections is especially critical to your well-being if you are an extrovert. Introverts undermine how critical socializing is to their wellness. Happy to spend time alone, introverts need time connecting with others the way we all need exercise to be healthy. Whether you gain energy from being alone or with others, social time is critical for well-being. Experiment with how much, and in which way, socializing optimizes your sense of happiness.

# Yoga Flow to Release Stress & Relax After Work

**1**

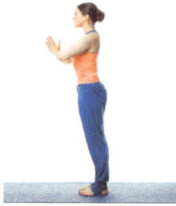

### Tadasana

-Press into all four
corners of the feet.
-Shoulders over hips.
-Lengthen tailbone
down and engage low
abs for a long spine.
-Hands to heart.

**2**

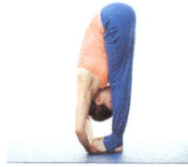

### Uttanasana

-Spread the arms out
as you fold over your
legs. Head drops last.
-Bring weight out of
the heels, pull abs in.
-Lift pelvic floor.
-Knees can be bent.

**3**

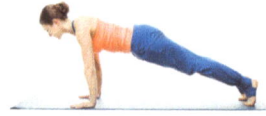

### Plank

-Bring shoulders over
wrists. Lift the pelvic
floor. Engage abs.
-Lengthen your
low back. Broaden
across the shoulders.
-Gaze soft.

**4**

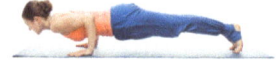

### Chaturanga

-Shift forward on your
toes. Stack shoul-
ders over wrists.
-Squeeze elbows
into the ribcage
as you lower down
in one line.
-Keep shoulders back.

**5**

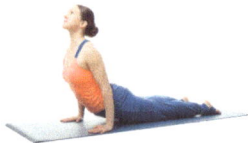

### Urdhva Mukha

-Lift the heart forward
and through the arms.
-Press into the tops of
the feet. Lift the legs.
-Roll shoulders back
and down the spine.
-Micro-bend the arms.

**6**

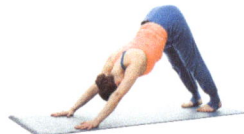

### Adho Mukha

-Spread fingers wide.
-Press the hips back as
push out of the arms.
-Lengthen the spine.
-Melt the heels down.
-Lift pelvic floor.
-Pull the belly inwards.

**7**

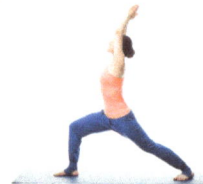

### Virabhadrasana I

-Ground the right foot
between the hands.
-Square the hips
forward. Ground
the edge of the
left foot down.
-Lift your arms up.
-Soften your ribs in.

**8**

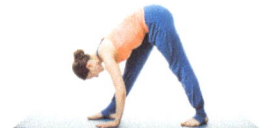

### Parsvottanasana

-Shorten your stance.
-Straighten both legs.
-Pull left hip back.
-Micro-bend left knee.
-Fold over your
left leg.
-Hands on floor or
blocks. Pull abs in.

Hold each pose for 3-5 deep, slow, even breaths with sound in and out the nose, creating a wave like sound with your breathing by constricting the back of the throat. Repeat the flow with the left leg and then relax in Shavasana for 5-10 minutes.

**9**

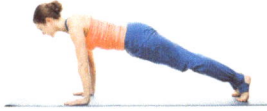

### Plank

-Bring shoulders over wrists. Lift the pelvic floor. Engage abs.
-Lengthen your low back. Broaden across the shoulders.
-Gaze soft.

**10**

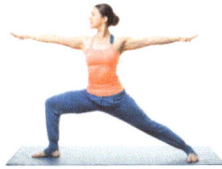

### Virabhadrasana II

-Ground the right foot between the hands.
-Pivot the left foot down and lift up.
-Stack shoulders over hips. Lift the heart.
-Pelvic floor lift.

**11**

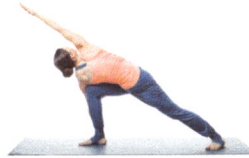

### Parivrtta Parsva-konasana

-Bring your left elbow to the outside of your right knee.
-Every inhale lengthen the spine. Exhale twist.
-Press left leg straight.

**12**

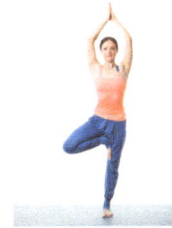

### Vrksasana

-Ground down into the left foot.
-Press the right foot to the inner thigh.
-Lift the arms, the heart. Relax shoulders.
-Engage pelvic floor.

**13**

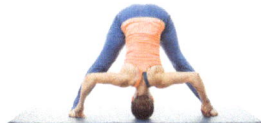

### Prasarita Padottanasana

-Grab your big toes.
-Fold forward in between your legs.
-Engage the legs.
-Lengthen the spine.
-Use the abs to fold.

**14**

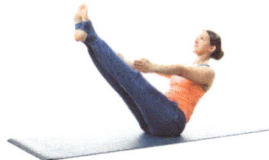

### Navasana

-Balance on sitting bones and lift legs.
-Hug legs together.
--Lengthen spine, engage your core.
-Draw shoulder blades on your back.

**15**

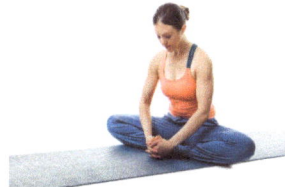

### Baddha Konasana

-Bring the soles of the feet together.
-Extend the spine.
-Press your knees down as your fold forward with a long spine.

**16**

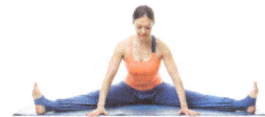

### Upavistha Konasana

-Open your legs wide.
- Press out through the heels. Lengthen spine.
-Roll inner thighs back and fold forward.
-Toes flexed up to sky.

**17**

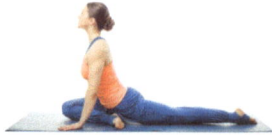

## Eka Pada Rajakapotasana

-Bend the right knee.
-Square the hips to the front of the mat. You can place a blanket under the hip here.
-Activate the left leg.

**18**

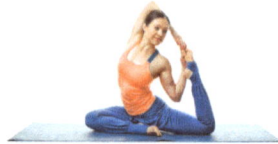

## Eka Pada Rajakapotasana

-Bend right knee in.
-Square the hips.
-Bend the left leg. Reach up and back with the right fingers for the left toes.

**19**

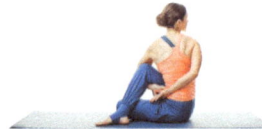

## Matsyendrasana

-Bend your left and right leg.
-Bring your right foot outside the left knee.
-Ground both sitting bones down.
-Arm to knee. Twist.

**20**

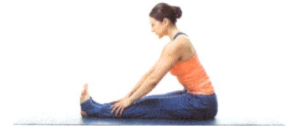

## Paschimottanasana

-Straighten both legs.
-Tilt pelvis forward.
-Press hamstrings into the mat. Long spine.
-Lift the pelvic floor; use the belly to pull you forward.

**21**

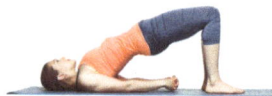

## Setu Bandha Sarvangasana

-Bring feet to the mat.
-Roll shoulders under. Clasp hands.
-Press into the feet. Pull inner thighs to mid line. Lift the hips

**22**

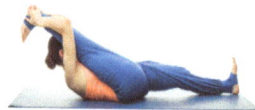

## Supta Padangusthasana

-Lie on your back.
-Bring your straight right leg into your chest while keeping the low back pressing into the mat.

**23**

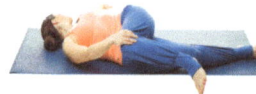

## Supta Matsyendrasana

-Lift the hips. Shift hips to right.
-Bend left knee and take it across the body.
-Stretch arms out.
-Look at left hand.

**24**

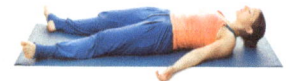

## Shavasana

-Straighten both legs.
-Roll onto your back. You can place a bolster under your knees.
-Pull the shoulder blades on your back.
-Relax everything.

# Sleeping

You can boost the quality of your sleep and your ability to fall asleep quickly. Start by going to bed at the same time each night.

Eliminate all digital electronics from the bedroom and make the room completely devoid of light when you go to sleep. Keep your bedroom cool. Avoid caffeine after lunchtime, alcohol after dinner time, and eating two hours before going to bed.

Go for a walk every day for at least ten minutes. Get out into daylight in the morning for at least a few minutes during the day and dim the lights a half hour before bed time. Ensure you've gotten enough high-quality fuel during the day; you need the energy to fall asleep and sleep through the night without being awakened by hunger pains. Release all worries and planning by making a habit of taking pen to paper and writing down what you need to get done the next days, tasks or appointments you don't want to forget, or worries plaguing the back of your mind. Taking pen to paper allows for a mind release before bed, freeing you to turn your thoughts off before sleep.

## PREPARE TO FALL INTO SLUMBER

With the jaws of time or fatigue clutching at your throat it can seem impossible to escape into a few minutes of restoration before bed. An evening yin sequence in silence or with calming meditation music for just ten minutes can ease you into blissful slumber. Taking time to be with any emotions arising before sleep in can rinse out any negative feelings from the day before they become imprinted in your body and mind. Few take time to be with themselves in this way.

Stopping and allowing emotions to arise and flow through you is a powerful way to un-cling from reaching for food, alcohol, drugs, drama, or digital distractions to push away what you don't want to feel. Repressed emotions lay just under the surface, waiting to boil up once the food is eaten, the glass of wine's effect fades, or the drama ends.

Meditation or yin yoga are two of the best ways to open up the self to feel and allow emotions to wash through you.

## SO WHAT IS YIN YOGA?

Introspective and meditative, in yin yoga you will hold each pose for around 3-5 minutes as you breathe deeply and rhythmically.

Surrender into the postures and allow healing and opening to happen in your deep tissues and fascia. Gentle surrender into the present moment allows the body to open and a wave of healing to wash over your body, mind, and spirit.

Settle into the pose, come to the point of sensation, and then become very still.

In a yin yoga sequence, it is settling into stillness and silence which has the healing effect on your body and mind. You will not only get a delicious deep stretch. Space and attention are opened for the body to release tension, stress, emotions, and energy blockages stored in the fascia.

The fascia is a net like web that surrounds all our muscles, tissues, and organs. Healthy fascia is fluid and dynamic like a newly spun spiderweb. Pain, lack of mobility and tension occurs when fascia becomes compacted and dense.

Re-hydrating and stimulating thick fascia to unravel and flow can provoke profound healing. Trauma and negative emotions like shame and fear can release through fascia work. You can discover a newfound fluidity

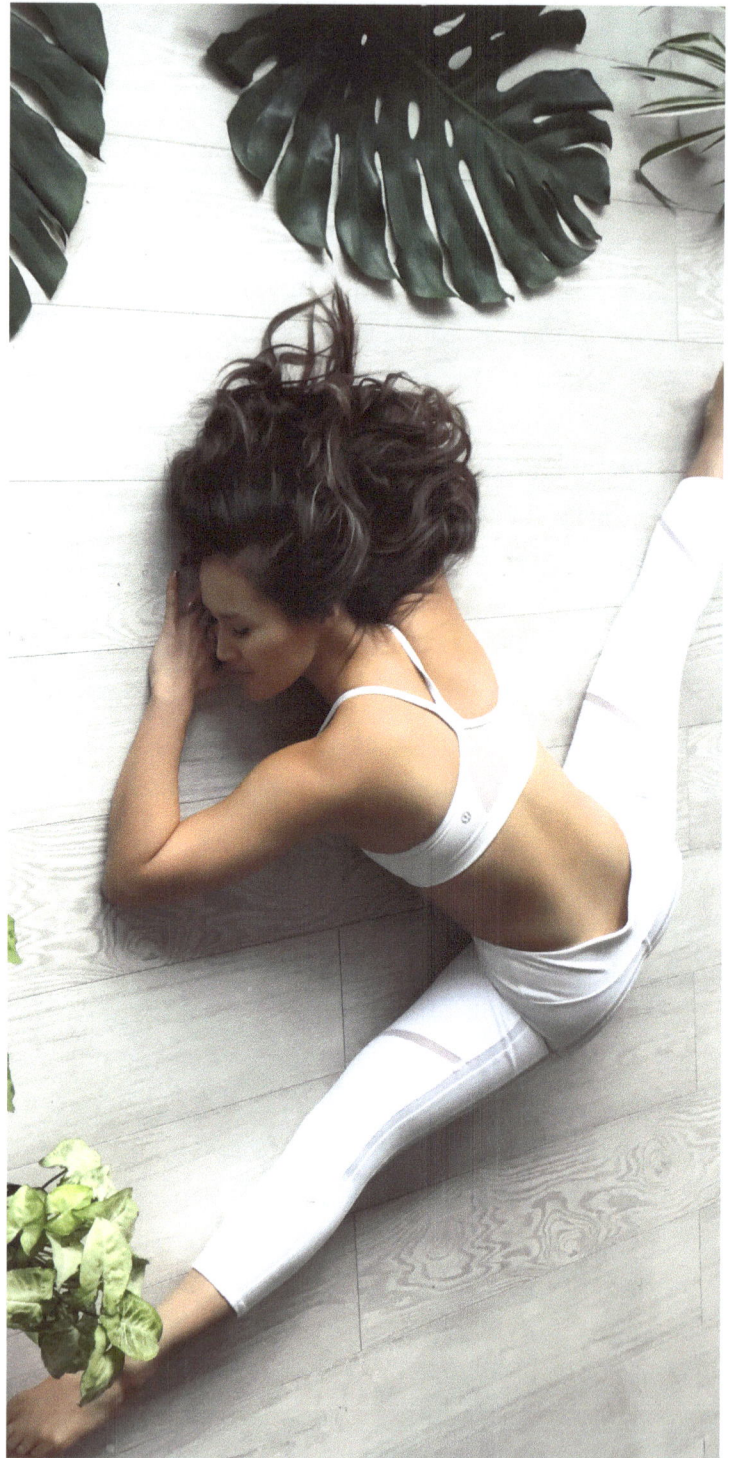

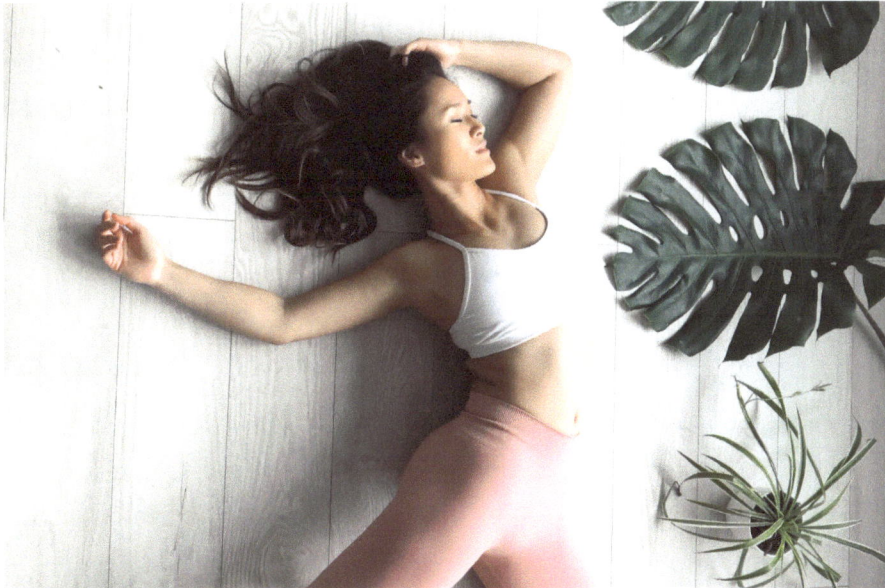

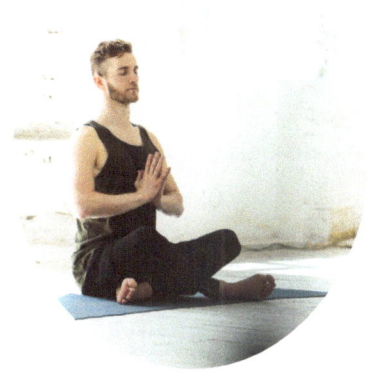

of movement and ease in the body. Yin yoga is one way of working on your fascia. Listen to your body and never sacrifice smooth, deep, even breathing through the nose. By breathing deeply from the belly and feeling your lungs expand in 360 degrees, you will be activating your parasympathetic nervous system, which will wash your body in repair and care treatment. Use the breath to anchor you to the present moment as emotions and thoughts float through and release.

## CREATE A REFUGE FOR REST

You can turn your bedroom into a haven for deep relaxation and sleep. Start by removing all high energy vibration elements from the room. Move any large mirror, television, desk, laptop, exercise equipment, and any work-related objects out of the bedroom.

Clear away clutter and introduce bedside tables on either side of your bed to introduce balance and harmony to your bedroom.

Add small lamps on the bedside tables to create soft lighting. Introduce high-quality sheets, and bedding in colors that uplift or soothe you. Light blues and greens provoke calm. White feels fresh, clean, and pure. You may be best served by a burst of color in the bedroom that lifts your spirit and prefer shades of purple, pink, yellow, or orange. Add artwork to the room that soothes or uplifts. Be careful to select art that sparks joy for you, or if you share your room, for your partner as well. Add in sensual or relaxing scents with a diffuser, candles, or a misting bottle.

Keeping a small misting bottle next to your bed filled with one ounce of water and six to ten drops of lavender essential oil. You can mist your pillow and bedding with the bottle before going to bed to improve your ability to fall asleep fast and deep.

Only use your bedroom as a refuge for rest and sleep. Doing so will train your body to associate with the bedroom and your bed as a place for deep relaxation, sensuality, and sleep.

## MIND REFRESH

Our minds can start to run on the same thoughts, creating deep grooves that restrict our ability to manifest what we desire. Imagine someone sitting next to you while you work on a project. Every few minutes they whisper something like, "this won't work you know," or "you're not smart enough." You try reasoning with them, convincing them, and even getting angry, so they leave you in peace to work. Nothing works. So you resign to ignore them. Many thoughts are unconscious and the average person thinks more than 40,000 thoughts a day.

Visualization, yoga nidra, hypnotherapy, and affirmations are not magic that will make all your dreams come true; yet they are tools that can create new mental grooves in your conscious mind and subconscious that support you, raise your energy, and boost your ability to forge forward and take action. You can listen to a hypnotherapy session before sleep each night to enter a state of deep relaxation while priming the subconscious to take positive action in an area of your choice. Free hypnotherapy, visualization, yoga nidra, and affirmation videos are available at Yoga with Heather on Youtube.

## AFFIRMATIONS

Our mind and subconscious can work against us. Dwindling energy, motivation, and a belief that manifesting our desires is impossible are the result. Affirmations must resonate with you to work and you need to believe in them. Creating your own affirmations in a voice memo on your phone and listening to them with earphones is the most effective. You can listen right before going to sleep and again during the day while doing chores or errands.

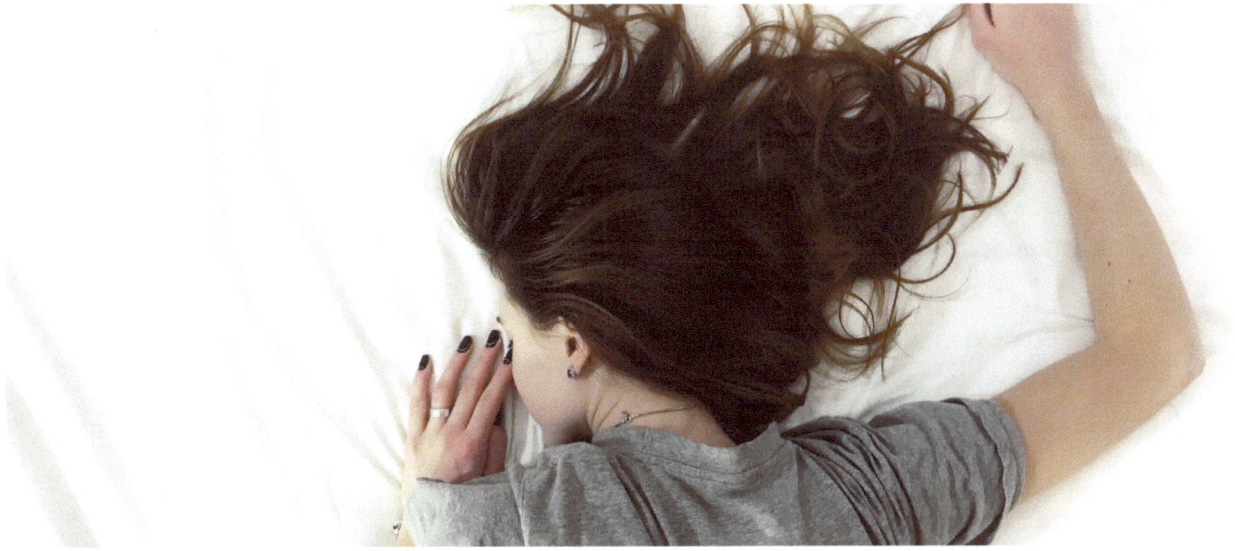

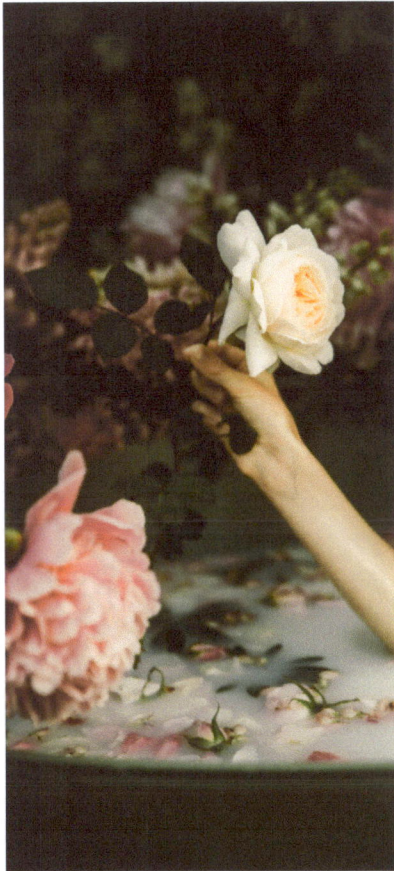

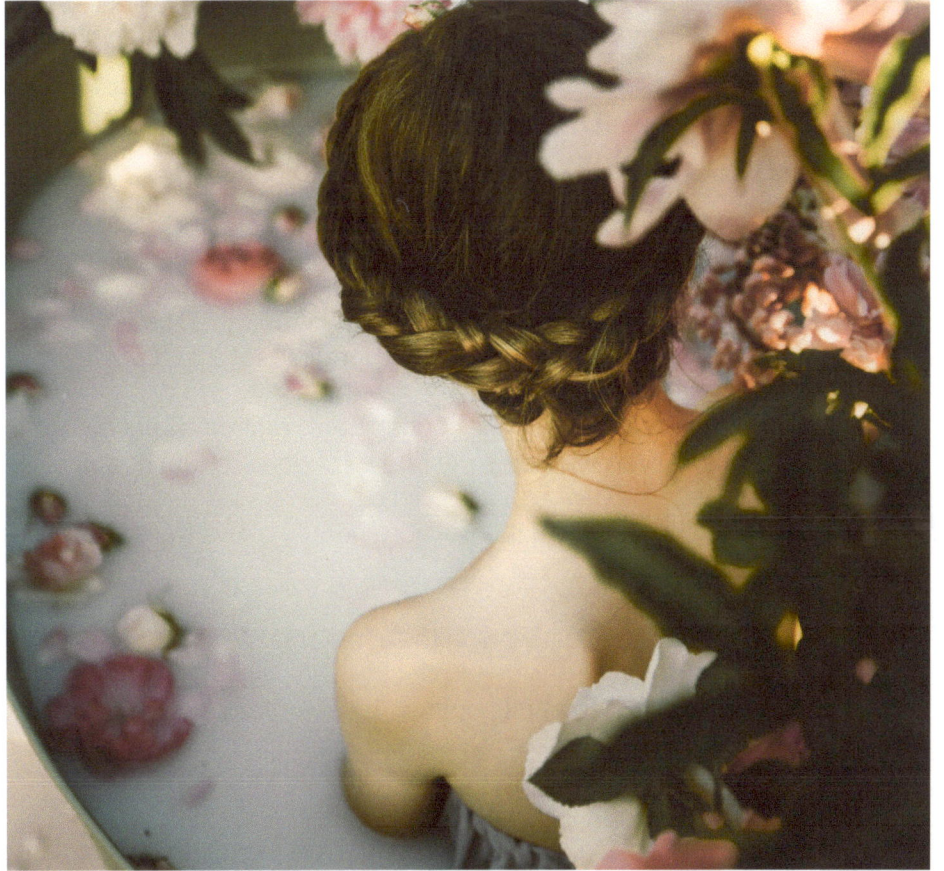

## STEPS TO CREATING YOUR AFFIRMATIONS

1. Begin healing trauma or pain first.
Affirmations are no replacement for working and releasing experiences and emotions.

2. Affirmations must feel like yours to work.

3. Use positive wording in the Present, without comparison to other points in time or others.

4. Feel that the affirmation exists now; experience the emotion of it being true.

5. Use your name. "I, Anna, do yoga and meditate every day."

6. Create affirmations you can believe and that resonate with you, or they will not work.

## AFFIRMATION IDEAS. BRAINSTORM YOUR OWN. FIND WHAT RESONATES WITH YOU. BELIEVE.

I think and talk about what I love and what brings me joy.

I focus my mind again and again on positive thoughts, feelings, and experiences. I focus on what I love and appreciate about everyone. I radiate love and positivity out into every relationship.

I listen to my body's needs for nourishment, rest, and movement. I love every cell of my body. I feel the inner aliveness inside my body. I choose to feel beautiful.

As love and stillness grow in me, more beauty glows from me. Well-being is expanding within me day by day.

I focus on giving my best work in this moment.

I get up and go to sleep at the same time everyday.

I do yoga and meditate everyday. I eat whole, fresh foods.

What I am feeling and giving is bringing everything into my life. I choose a higher vibration.

Wellness wants me. Joy wants me. Peace wants me.

Gratitude to the great multiplier in my life. I give thanks.

I imagine all the things that can go RIGHT.

There is enough for everyone, including me. I have everything I need. I like money and use it well.

I am worthy of love, wellness, abundance, peace, joy. Love, wellness, abundance, peace, joy flows to me.

I have ever renewing energy and love flowing through me.

I spend time in nature and open to the beauty and stillness.

Everyday I am becoming more successful through action. It is not what I do, but how I do what I do which determines fulfilling my desire.

A wave of creativity is flowing through me into my work.

I am fearless. I am immune to criticism. I am above and below no one. I feel no higher, nor lower, than anyone. I need no outside validation.

I am building an environment and life around me I love. I radiate love and light out to others and the world.

My body is an energy field of radiant health and vitality.

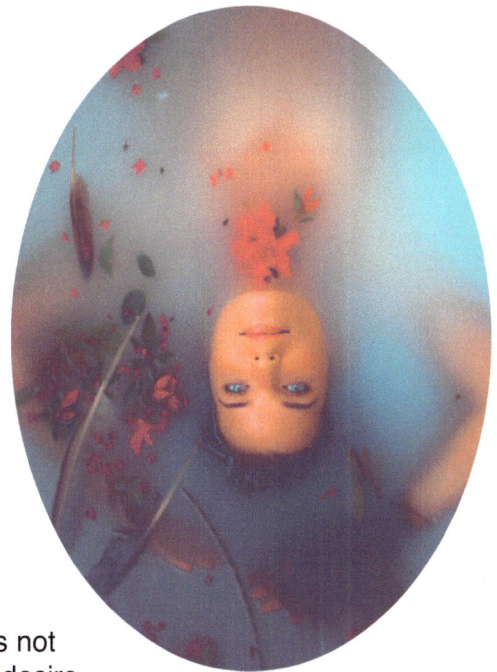

## BEFORE BED VISUALIZATION

The first step is to know your desire. Take at least five minutes to sit in a quiet place. So many of us focus on what is 'out there' that needs changing instead of realizing the power of changing what is 'in here', No matter what our life situation, we can change how we interact with others and find rest within ourselves. Close your eyes and place a hand over your heart and another over your solar plexus or belly. Envision how you want to show up in the world and feel inwardly.

Perhaps you see yourself glowing with health, serenity, fulfillment, and lightheartedness. Or you exude quiet steel strength, character, confidence, and kindness as you move through your days. How do you interact with other people? Now shift your focus to visualizing what a fulfilling life of happiness would be for you. What work are you doing? How do you give of yourself and how are your close relationships? How do you spend your working and free hours?

Take out a pen and paper and write down who you want to be and the life you want to be living. Next, analyze where you are and what you need to do to transform your life. Work within your sphere of influence. The gap between now and your vision may appear like a canyon you can never cross. Allow hope. Write down just three steps you can begin taking right away to start your evolution journey. You can record your visualization and listen to it right before bed. Or place your visualization notes in your bedside drawer. Take it out right before bed every night and read it through. Then close your eyes and visualize the person and life you want to manifest. Next, see yourself taking the three active steps toward making the vision a reality the next day. Release the vision and draw your attention to the breath. On each inhalation visualize golden light streaming up your feet, through your legs, torso, arms, to your fingertips, up your spine to the crown of your head.

On your exhalation feel the golden light flow back down through every inch of your body and back to the soles of your feet. Take ten deep, slow breaths continuing to visualize the flow of golden light up and down your body. Grounding into the body with our awareness before sleep can quiet your mind, release your mind from running away in mental movies or worry, and ease you gently into deep regenerative sleep.

## BODY LOVE & BEAUTY

Do you love your body? Time to start. Say to your body each night while brushing your teeth: Body, body, body, I LOVE you. Repeat three times. You may feel silly. Do it anyway. Now allow yourself to feel attractive, sexy, beautiful, pretty, or any other word that resonates with you. Instead of fixating on the outward appearance, turn your attention to the inner body. How well do you feel? Do you feel good? Allow this inner well-being to be linked with how beautiful you feel. Your inner light of well-being is what is glowing out beauty from you.

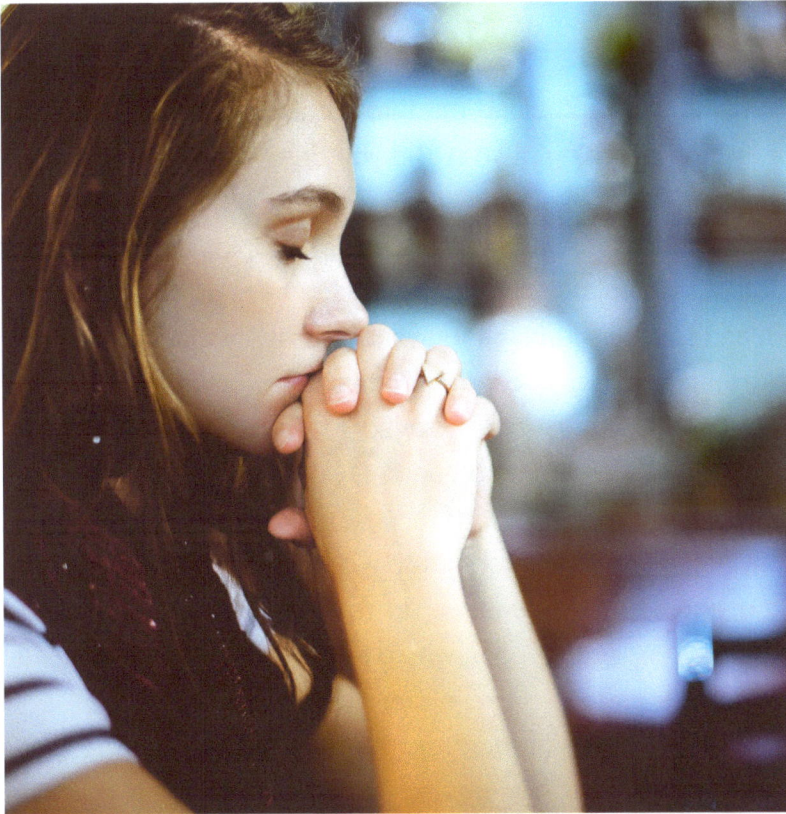

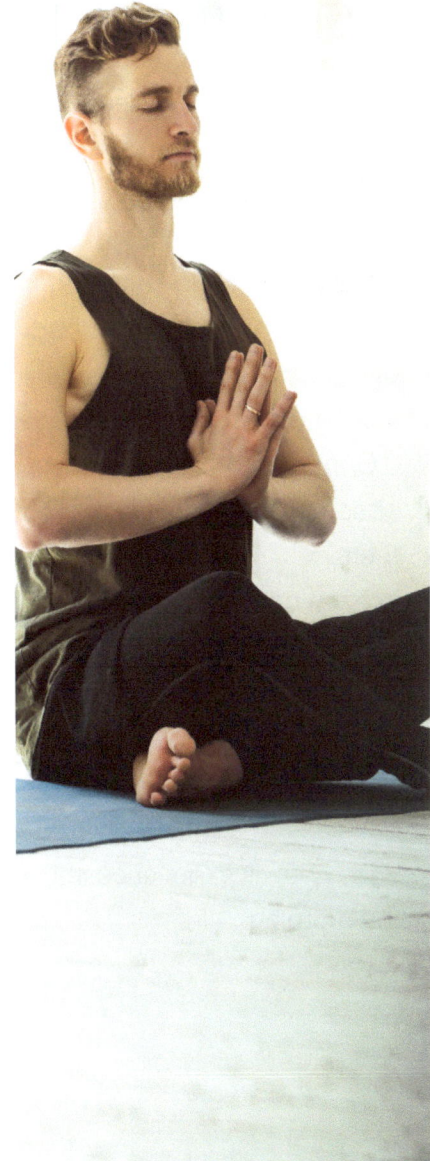

## PRAYING OR SENDING LIGHT

Prayer and energy are powerful. You can make a difference. You can send healing or loving light energy to people, situations, and yourself before you fall asleep every night. If you pray for people or situations, then pray: "May the best thing happen." Or "May the best outcome prevail for everyone involved." Feel love flowing out from your heart.

*"If you are depressed you are living in the past. If you are anxious you are living in the future. If you are at peace you are living in the present." - Lao Tzu*

## INSOMNIA

If you wake up in the middle of the night and can't sleep run through a checklist. Did you eat enough during the day? Is worry or anxiety clutching at you? Did you drink caffeine in the afternoon or evening? Did you drink any alcohol before bedtime? Did you spend time out in the fresh air? Did you exercise? Did you take a multivitamin and a magnesium supplement? Changing your daily life can quickly alleviate future insomnia.

Don't panic if you can't wind down and fall asleep at night or wake up in the middle of the night and can't fall back asleep. First, make yourself a cup of chamomile tea. Chamomile tea calms the nervous system and settles the nerves. Next, put on some cozy socks and clothes, so you feel warm and comfortable. Roll out your yoga mat or find a soft carpet. Spray some lavender oil or add three drops to hand lotion to soothe and relax you.

Doing some Yin Yoga and then unwinding into even more profound relaxation with a Yoga Nidra session will allow your body, mind, and soul to find rest. In Yin Yoga, especially in the middle of the night when you are all alone, you will open up space where repressed emotions can surface and dissolve. Be courageous.

Continue to breathe and be with whatever arises in the present moment. Become the silent observer watching any thoughts or emotions that arise without identifying or getting caught up in them. You may find that no strong feelings arise, and this is okay too. Continue to breathe deeply in each pose and know that the work is being done on a subconscious level.

In Yoga Nidra, you will be guided into a state of 'yogic sleep' in which you bring your attention to each part of the body as you breathe slowly and deeply. Deep breathing and relaxing each part of the body activates the parasympathetic nervous system, which allows your body to rest and repair. You may become sleepy after the Yin and Yoga Nidra sessions and easily drift into slumber. Or, you may rest quietly, drawing your attention over and over again to your breath. Either way, you will experience rejuvenation and feel calmer, more balanced, and full of more energy in the morning.

# YIN YOGA TO WIND DOWN FOR SLEEP

**Hold each pose for THREE MINUTES.  Breathe with sound in and out the nose, creating a wave like sound with your breathing by constricting the back of the throat.**

**1**

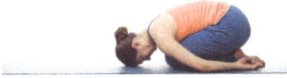

### Child's Pose

-Bring your feet together, open your knees, hips to heels, melt your forehead to the floor. -Allow the back body to soften. Breathe.

**2**

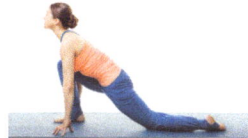

### Dragon Pose

-Right knee over ankle. -Lower left knee to the mat. -Fingertips frame the foot or lift skyward. -Sink the hips. -Repeat on left side.

**3**

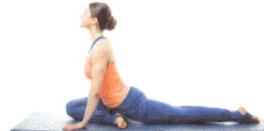

### Upward Swan Pose

-Bend the right knee. -Square the hips to the front of the mat. You can place a blanket under the hip here. -Repeat on left side.

**4**

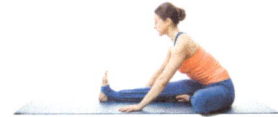

### Janu Sirsasana

-Square your hips forward as your bring the left foot to the inside of the right thigh. -Lengthen the spine. -Use the belly to fold. -Repeat on left side.

**5**

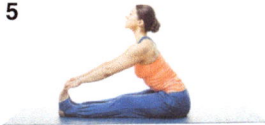

### Caterpillar Pose

-Straighten both legs. -Tilt pelvis forward. -Press hamstrings into the mat. Long spine. -Lift the pelvic floor; use the belly to pull you forward.

**6**

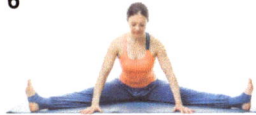

### Dragon Fly Pose

-Open your legs wide. - Press out through the heels. -Lengthen spine. -Roll inner thighs back and fold forward slowly, breathing deeply. -Toes flexed up to sky.

**7**

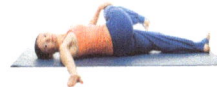

### Supta Matsyendrasana

-Lift the hips. Shift hips to right. -Bend right knee and take it across the body. -Look at left hand. -Repeat on left side.

**8**

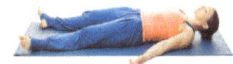

### Shavasana

-Straighten both legs. -Roll  onto your back. You can place a bolster under your knees. -Pull the shoulder blades on your back. -Relax everything. -Melt into the mat.

# Ayurveda

## What is your AYURVEDA dosha body type?

We are all born with a certain Prakriti, or constitution. Each person is a combination of all three doshas. Kapha grounds and calms us, giving us structure and stability as it opens us to patience and love. Pitta provides us with metabolism, fire for courage, discipline, willpower, competition, and change. Vata gives us movement to create, express, be flexible and vivacious.

The original nature we are born with has one predominant dosha, though some individuals have two doshas in equal portion. For example, this manifests as a similar combination of Vata and Pitta or Pitta and Kapha.

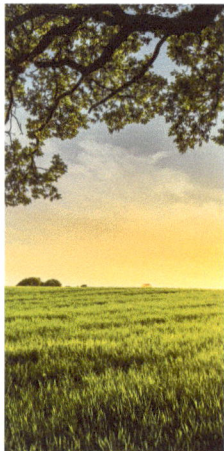 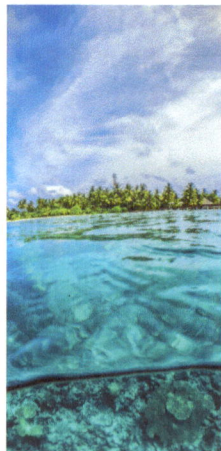 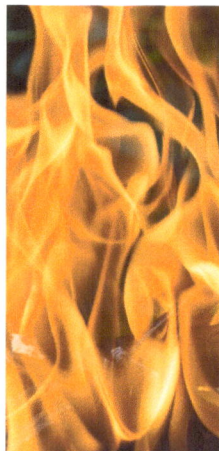 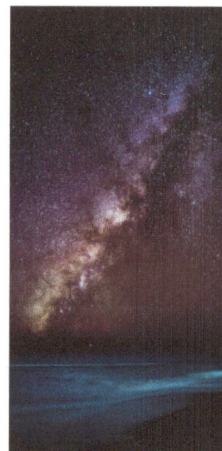 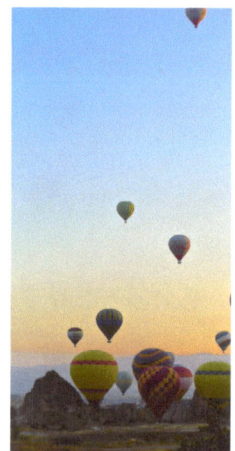

| EARTH | WATER | FIRE | SPACE | AIR |

# WHAT IS YOUR DOSHA BODY TYPE?

## VATA BODY TYPE

People with a predominance of VATA in their bodies are small boned, lean, slow to gain weight, and can experience creaking or cracking joints. Vatas have energy that fluctuates, coming in bright bursts of activity. A VATA body type gets cold easily, has dry skin and hair, and can be challenged with difficulty falling or staying asleep, bloating, constipation, and too much weight loss when out of balance.

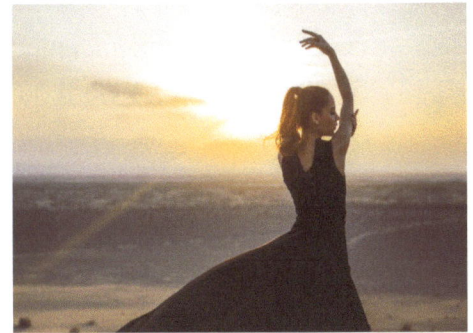

## PITTA BODY TYPE

People with a predominance of PITTA in their bodies can gain muscle easily, gain or lose weight easily, and are medium built. High in energy and fire, PITTAs need exercise to burn off some of their internal heat so they can cool and calm down. PITTAs need regular meals; they become irritable if they miss lunch. A PITTA body type has oily skin and soft hair and gets too hot and sweats easily. Pitta can be challenged with too much stomach acidity causing heartburn, ulcers, or diarrhea when out of balance, as well as acne, skin rashes, and inflammation.

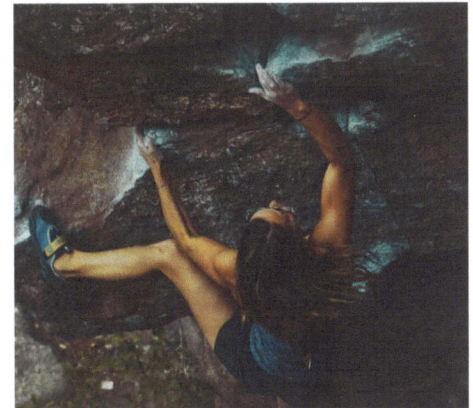

## KAPHA BODY TYPE

People with a predominance of KAPHA in their bodies have strength and stamina, bigger bones, round faces, thick hair, full, soft lips, moist, cool, soft skin, cold, clammy hands, and feet. A KAPHA body type gains weight easily and loses weight with difficulty. While the sluggish metabolism of a KAPHA body type is a challenge for them, KAPHAs tend to age beautifully due to their moist, supple skin.

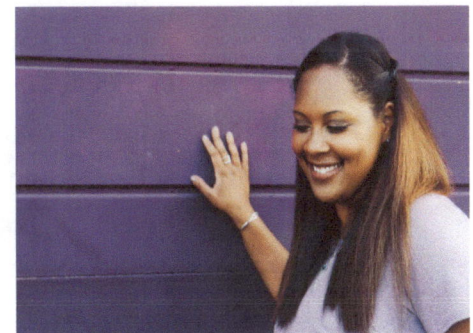

# WHAT IS YOUR DOSHA MIND TYPE?

## VATA MIND TYPE

People with a predominance of Vata in their mind are energetic, imaginative, creative, artistic, innovative thinkers, enthusiastic, lively, and brilliant communicators who like change and variety. Although VATAs learn quickly, they also forget quickly. VATAs love constant change and generally are working on a number of projects at the same time. When they slip out of balance VATAs become spacey; they lose their focus and ability to make decisions and all the balls they are juggling begin to fall. Suddenly they are overwhelmed and confused.

Under stress, VATAs inherent tendency is to become flighty, sleepless, fearful, anxious, insecure, or worried.

## PITTA MIND TYPE

People with a predominance of PITTA in their mind enjoy learning new things, are ambitious, of keen intellect, joyful, and disciplined, with a fire to go after goals and get a job done right. PITTAs tend towards leadership as they like working in a team, are excellent communicators who love to convince, thrive in competition, and like to solve problems. Perfectionists, PITTAs can be hypercritical of themselves and others and learn new things.

Under stress PITTAs instinctive tendency is to snap at others around them, become aggressive, resentful, jealous, controlling, or erupt like a volcano.

## KAPHA MIND TYPE

People with a predominance of KAPHA in their mind have a grounded, stable, easy-going personality and are stress resilient, slow to anger, and loyal. Good listeners, methodical workers, supportive and dependable, KAPHAS make great team members. KAPHAs may not learn as fast as others, but once they learn it, their long-term memory is excellent. KAPHAs find solace in a routine and staying in their comfort zone. Reliable and patient, KAPHA likes to support and are often humorous and good-natured.

Under stress KAPHAs have instinctive tendency to lose their motivation and forward momentum; they become sad, depressed, unhealthily attached, lethargic, withdrawn, or reclusive.

## MOVING INTO BALANCE

Now that you know your unique constitutional dosha type, it is time to analyze your internal and external environment. Lifestyle and dietary choices can support your radiant energy and vitality or cause mental and bodily imbalances and illness. Imbalance can occur in your doshas when you live contrary to your birth constitution, by making wrong choices for YOU in regards to your diet, environment, occupation, exercise, thoughts, actions, emotions, sensory inputs, self-care, or stimulation levels.

Understanding your dosha type means you can discover which steps are right for YOU to take to regain your equilibrium and find your way back to homeostasis for vibrant health and well-being.

Different types will require different well-being action steps to find balance, vitality, health. For example, whereas a predominant VATA person in both mind and body will thrive on a routine to ground, calm, and nourish, a predominant KAPHA person in body and mind will do the best by adding change and spice into their daily life.

Be aware that your balance of doshas can be different for your body and mind. Whereas I am a Vata in body, I am a dualistic Pitta in mind. The result is that I need to look to how to balance Vata physically and Vata Pitta mentally to bring myself into balance. It is rare that we can attain a perfect balance all the time. For instance, a Vata type needs to stay up late to celebrate a wedding even though he is best served by going to bed at the same time every night. The objective is to know which actions to take to bring ourselves physically and mentally back into balance.

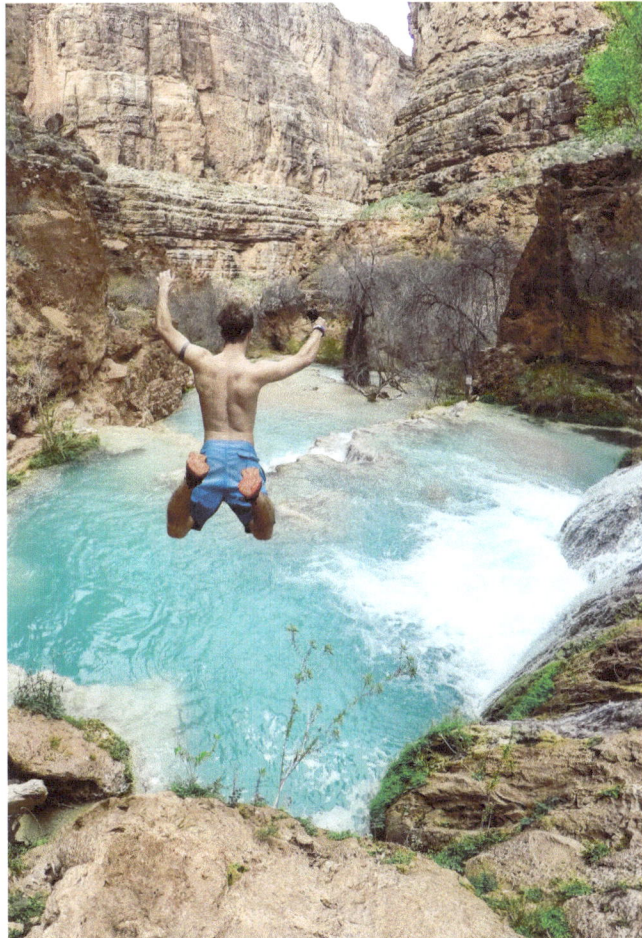

## Ways to Balance VATA

### Grounding, Warming, Moisturizing, Stability, and Routine

-Create and follow a daily routine and be sure to eat at regular meal times and wake up at the same time every day.
   Hydrate throughout the day.

-Meditate each morning and evening for twenty minutes. Begin your day with yoga or tai chi when kapha energy is at its peak.

-Include in your daily self-care an oil massage after your shower or bath. Take almond, olive, or another natural, organic oil into your palm. Rub in long strokes over your muscles and in circular movements over joints and your belly.

-Spend time each day in a peaceful environment and in nature.

-Go to bed before ten pm and get at least eight hours of sleep. Wake up at the same time daily.

-Avoid or moderate your intake of coffee, black tea, cigarettes, and alcohol. Need a comfort or reward replacement? Try a cup of chamomile tea or a mug of warm milk with one or a combination of the following: cinnamon, cardamom, nutmeg, ginger, grated vanilla.

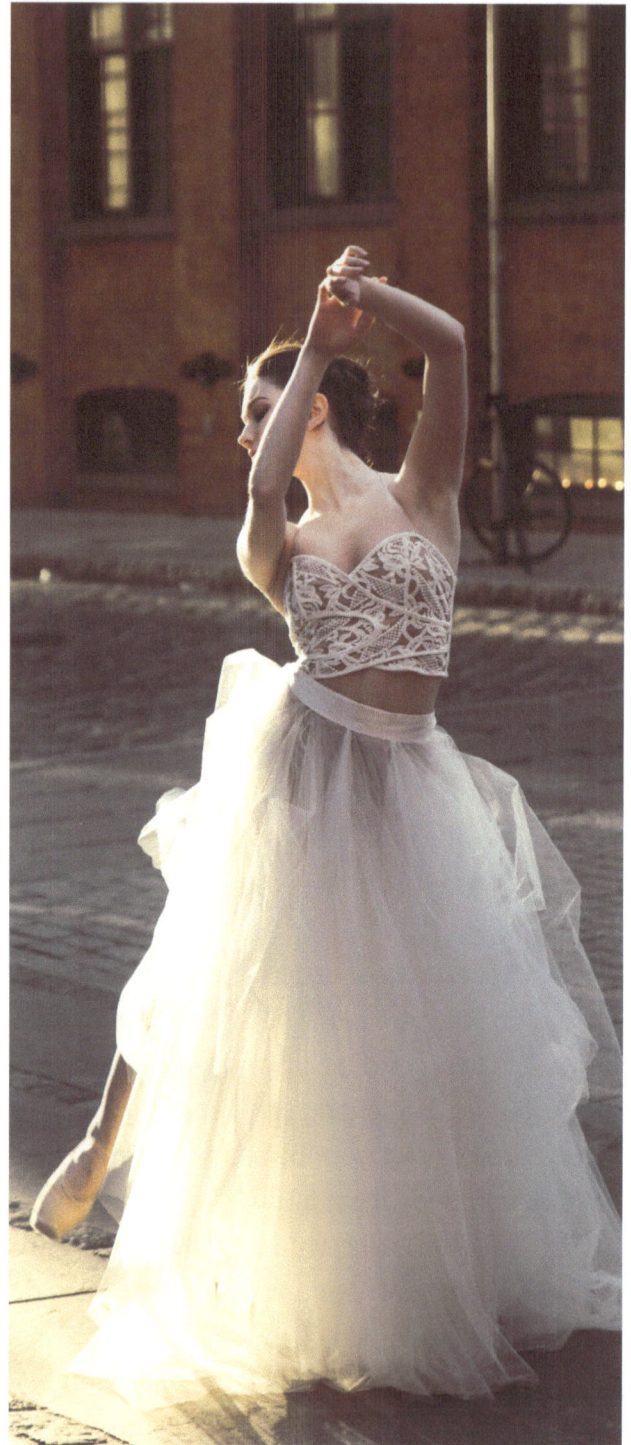

-Eat Vata-balancing foods, such as potatoes, sweet potatoes, other veggies grown in the earth, spices, such as cinnamon, cardamom, turmeric, stews, curries, soups, and oatmeal.

-Take one to five minutes before each meal to 'get earthy' by laying flat on the floor, or by breathing in deeply and slowly to the count of three and exhaling to the count of six. While eating turn off and put away all electronics.

-Complete a Yin Yoga class or Yoga Nidra weekly and walk barefoot in the grass to ground your energy.

-Use breathing techniques to slow down the breath.

## Ways to Balance PITTA

### Cooling, Nourishing, Calming, Moderation

-Begin your day with high-intensity exercise to burn off some of the internal fire to calm and balance.

Follow your training with a few minutes of calming physical activity, such as tai chi, restorative yoga, or yin yoga, and a ten minute meditation.

-Avoid or moderate your intake of coffee, black tea, cigarettes, and alcohol. Need a comfort or reward replacement?

Try a cup of mint or fennel tea, both of which are cooling, or make up a pitcher of water with sliced cucumbers.

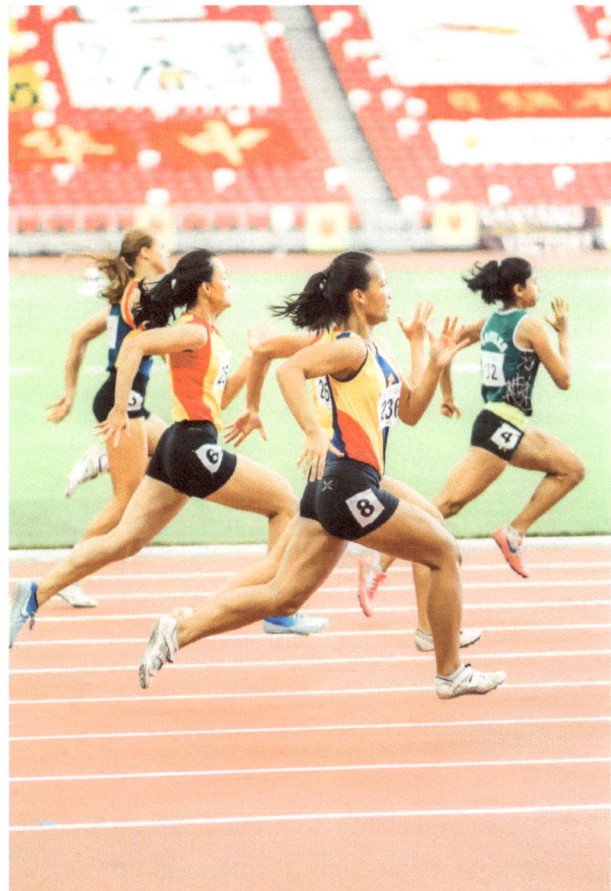

141

-Don't skip meals, which will cause you to become irritable and uneasy.

-Take one to five minutes before each meal to chill and cool your inner fire by folding forward, clasping opposite elbows, and hanging for a few moments. Another option is to breathe in deeply and slowly to the count of three and exhale to the count of six for two minutes. While eating turn off all electronics.

-Eat Pitta-balancing foods, such as summer foods like leafy greens, mint, cucumbers, berries, raw foods, rice, whole grains, and coconut oil.

-Engage in at least one calming activity that isn't competitive, liking gardening, walking in the woods, or painting. Focus on the process, instead of on the end goal or result.

- Pittas tend towards perfectionism, criticism, over competitiveness, and fire. Take a break of a few minutes, multiple times a day to move, breathe deeply and slowly, regain your suppleness, calm, reconnect with joy, get outside, and nourish your body, mind, and soul.

## Ways to Balance KAPHA

## Stimulating, Drying, Warming, Stimulating, Moving

-Drink a cup of hot water with freshly squeezed lemon to wake up your sluggish digestion first thing in the morning.

-Begin your day with stimulating exercise, such as a brisk walk or run outside, interval training, or a vinyasa or power yoga flow. Finish with one to two minutes of breath of fire, which is a rapid exhalation of the breath through the nose. Keep the mouth closed and on each fast exhale, pull the belly button in toward the spine and upwards. The inhale is passive. Breath of fire will stimulate digestion, heat, and inner drive.

-Eat Kapha-balancing foods, such as steamed vegetables, quinoa, amaranth, and stimulating spices such as cayenne pepper and turmeric. Eat dairy and sweets in tiny amounts.

-Take one to five minutes before each meal to open the heart by sitting tall, grounding down into the sitting bones, placing your fingertips behind you, and lifting the heart up to the sky for ten breaths. How are you feeling? Are you going to eat to nourish your body, or is it your mind or soul that needs nourishing? Give comfort to yourself in non-food ways if you are reaching for food to uplift your mood.

-Take a walk outside in the fresh air after every meal.

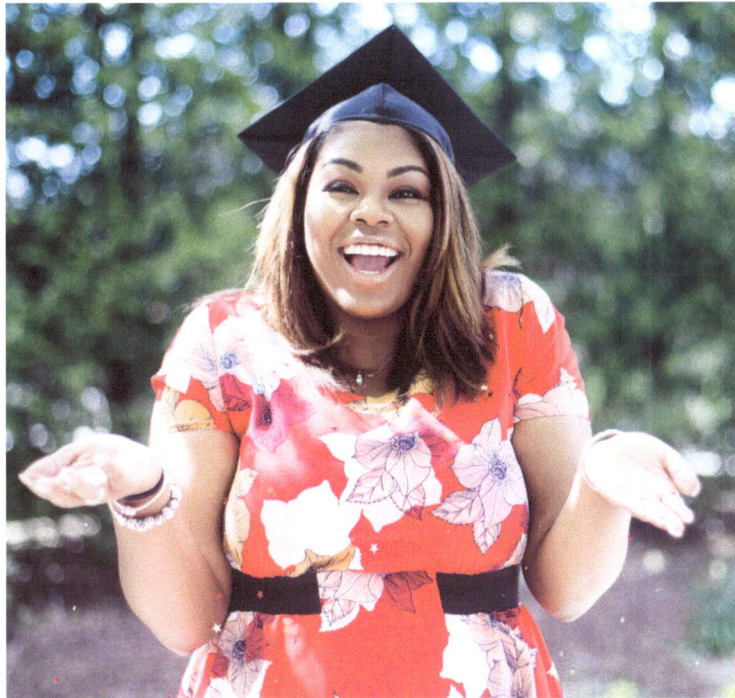

-Kaphas love luxury, comfort, and predictability, so balance your dosha by adding adventure, fasting one morning a week, and scheduling in stimulating activities that push you outside your physical and mental comfort zones.

-Meditate once a day for twenty minutes and follow with introspection and journaling. Kaphas are natural supporters with a tendency to suppress negative emotions. Take time to let go of these negative emotions with yoga, journaling, meditating, prayer, time in nature, or talking to a loved one. Find your inner spaciousness, and channel your intuition, so you know the difference between being kind and letting yourself be taken advantage of quickly.

-Go to bed before ten pm and rise early. Avoid naps.

*"What you think, you become. What you feel, you attract. What you imagine, you create." - Buddha*

# Yoga Flow to BALANCE VATA

**1**

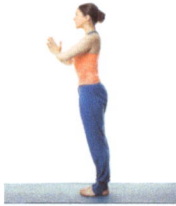

### Tadasana

-Press into all four
corners of the feet.
-Shoulders over hips.
-Lengthen tailbone
down and engage low
abs for a long spine.
-Hands to heart.

**2**

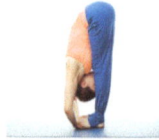

### Uttanasana

-Spread the arms out
as you fold over your
legs. Head drops last.
-Bring weight out of
the heels, pull abs in.
-Lift pelvic floor.
-Knees can be bent.

**3**

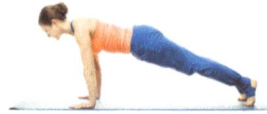

### Plank

-Bring shoulders over
wrists. Lift the pelvic
floor. Engage abs.
-Lengthen your
low back. Broaden
across the shoulders.
-Gaze soft.

**4**

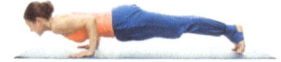

### Chaturanga

-Shift forward on your
toes. Stack shoul-
ders over wrists.
-Squeeze elbows
in to the ribcage as
you lower down.
-Keep shoulders back.

**5**

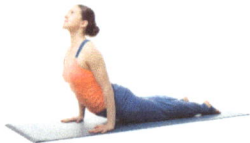

### Urdhva Mukha

-Lift the heart forward
and through the arms.
-Press into the tops of
the feet. Lift the legs.
-Roll shoulders back
and down the spine.
-Micro-bend the arms.

**6**

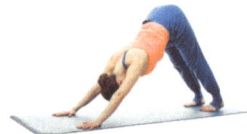

### Adho Mukha

-Spread fingers wide.
-Press the hips
back as you push
out of the arms.
-Lengthen the spine.
-Melt the heels down.
-Pull the belly inwards.

**7**

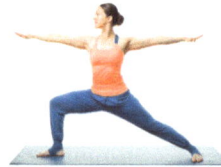

### Virabhadrasana II

-Ground the right foot
between the hands.
-Pivot the left foot
down and lift up.
-Stack shoulders over
hips. Lift the heart.
-Pelvic floor lift.

**8**

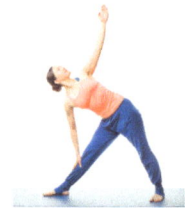

### Trikonasana

-Straighten the leg.
-Pull the right
hip back.
-Extend the side body.
-Reach forward. Re-
lease the right hand
to your shin or block.
-Extend left arm up.

Hold each pose for 3-5 deep, slow, even breaths with sound in and out the nose, creating a wave like sound with your breathing by constricting the back of the throat. Repeat the flow with the left leg and then relax in Shavasana for 5-10 minutes.

**9**

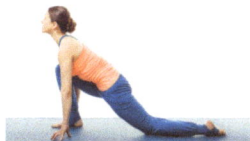

### Anjaneyasana

-Right knee over ankle.
-Lower left knee to the mat. Square hips.
-Fingertips frame the foot or lift skyward.
-Sink the hips.

**10**

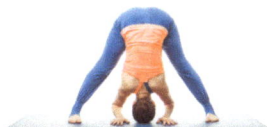

### Prasarita Padottanasana

-Fold forward.
-Hands between feet.
-Engage the legs.
-Lengthen the spine.
-Use the abs to fold.

**11**

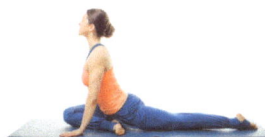

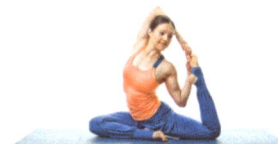

### Eka Pada Rajakapotasana

-Bend the right knee.
-Square the hips to the front of the mat. You can place a blanket under the hip here.
-Activate the left leg.

**12**

### Eka Pada Rajakapotasana

-Bend right knee in.
-Square the hips.
-Bend the left leg. Reach up and back with the right fingers for the left toes.

**13**

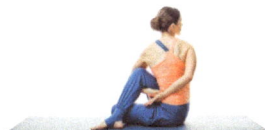

### Matsyendrasana

-Bend your left and right leg.
-Bring your right foot outside the left knee.
-Ground both sitting bones down.
-Arm to knee. Twist.

**14**

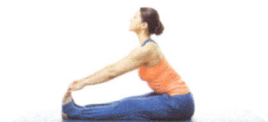

### Paschimottanasana

-Straighten both legs.
-Tilt pelvis forward.
-Press hamstrings into the mat. Long spine.
-Lift the pelvic floor; use the belly to pull you forward.

**15**

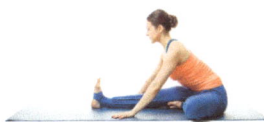

### Janu Sirsasana

-Square your hips forward as your bring the left foot to the inside of the right thigh.
-Lengthen the spine.
-Use the belly to fold you forward.

**16**

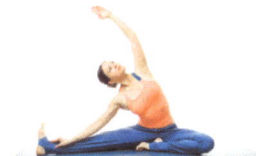

### Parivrtta Upavistha

-Lift your left arm up and over your right ear.
-Right elbow on your thigh or floor.
-Stretch the side body.
-Revolve heart up.

**17**

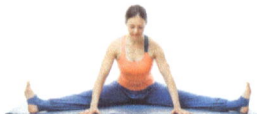

## Upavistha Konasana

-Open your legs wide.
- Press out through the heels. Lengthen spine.
-Roll inner thighs back and fold forward.
-Toes flexed up to sky.

**18**

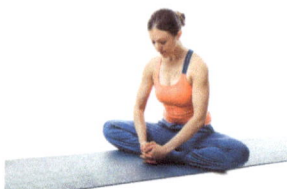

## Baddha Konasana

-Bring the soles of the feet together.
-Open feet like a book
-Extend the spine.
-Press your knees down as your fold forward with a long spine.

**19**

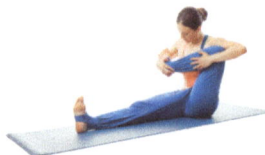

## Seated Eka Pada Rajakapotasana

-Straighten the right leg. Bend the left leg. Bring the left foot to the crook of the right elbow. Pull to chest.
-Sit up taller.

**20**

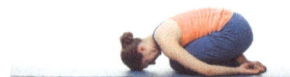

## Balasana

-Bring your feet together, open your knees, hips to heels, melt your forehead to the floor.
-Allow the back body to soften. Breathe.

**21**

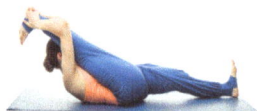

## Supta Padangusthasana

-Lie on your back.
-Bring your straight right leg into your chest while keeping the low back pressing into the mat.

**22**

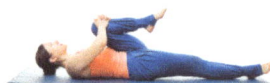

## Knee to Chest

-Grab your left knee and pull it into your chest.
-Press the low back into the floor.
-Relax your shoulders away from your ears.

**23**

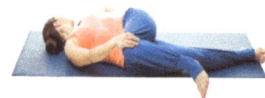

## Supta Matsyendrasana

-Lift the hips. Shift hips to right.
-Bend left knee and take it across the body.
-Stretch arms out.
-Look at left hand.

**24**

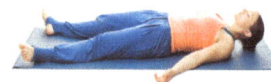

## Shavasana

-Straighten both legs.
-Roll onto your back. You can place a bolster under your knees.
-Pull the shoulder blades on your back.
-Relax everything.

# Yoga Flow to BALANCE PITTA

**1**

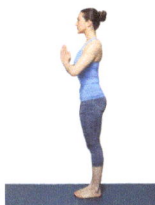

### Tadasana

-Press into all four
corners of the feet.
-Shoulders over hips.
-Lengthen tailbone
down and engage low
abs for a long spine.
-Hands to heart.

**2**

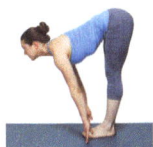

### Ardha Uttanasana

-Spread the arms out
as you fold over your
legs. Head drops last.
-Inhale, lengthen, look
forward, pull abs in.
-Lift pelvic floor.
-Fold over your legs.

**3**

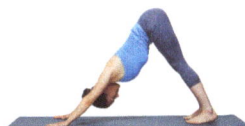

### Adho Mukha

-Spread fingers wide.
-Press the hips back
-Lengthen the spine.
-Melt the heels down.
-Lift pelvic floor.
-Pull the belly inwards.

**4**

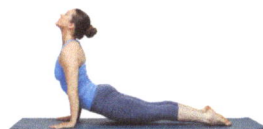

### Urdhva Mukha

-Lift the heart forward
and through the arms.
-Press into the tops of
the feet. Lift the legs.
-Roll shoulders back
and down the spine.
-Micro-bend the arms.

**5**

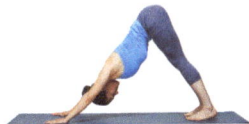

### Adho Mukha

-Press the hips
back as you push
out of the arms.
-Lengthen the spine.
-Melt the heels down.
-Lift pelvic floor.
-Pull the belly inwards.

**6**

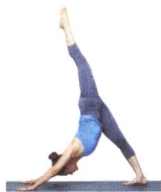

### Eka Pada Adho Mukha

-Lengthen the spine.
-Lift pelvic floor as
you hollow the belly.
-Abs engaged as you
lift the left leg up to
the sky. Square hips.

**7**

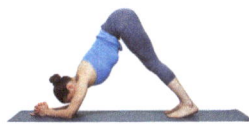

### Prep Pincha Mayurasana

-Ground forearms
shoulder width apart.
-Curl toes under.
Straighten the legs.
-Lift one leg up and
then the other.

**8**

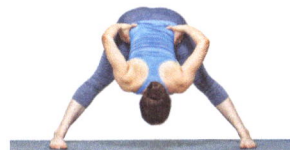

### Prasarita Padottanasana

-Hands to hips.
-Fold forward in
between your legs.
-Engage the legs.
-Lengthen the spine.
-Use the abs to fold.

Hold each pose for 3-5 deep, slow, even breaths with sound in and out the nose, creating a wave like sound with your breathing by constricting the back of the throat. Repeat the flow with the right leg and then relax in Shavasana for 5-10 minutes.

**9**

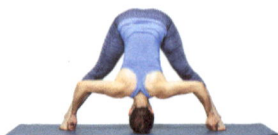

### Prasarita Padottanasana

-Grab your big toes.
-Fold forward in between your legs.
-Engage the legs.
-Lengthen the spine.
-Use the abs to fold.

**10**

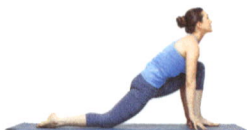

### Anjaneyasana

-Left knee over ankle.
-Lower right knee to the mat. Square hips.
-Fingertips frame the foot or lift skyward.
-Lengthen the spine.
-Sink the hips.

**11**

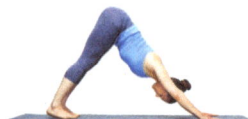

### Adho Mukha

-Spread fingers wide.
-Press the hips back.
-Lengthen the spine.
-Melt the heels down.
-Lift pelvic floor.
-Pull the belly inwards.

**12**

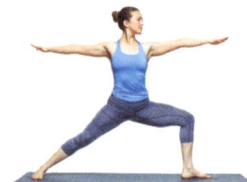

### Virabhadrasana II

-Ground the left foot between the hands.
-Pivot the right foot down and lift up.
-Stack shoulders over hips. Lift the heart.
-Lift pelvic floor.

**13**

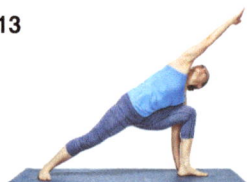

### Parsvakonasana

-Left knee over left ankle. Draw the right arm over the right ear.
-Roll left hip under.
-Stretch from the outer edge of the right foot up through the fingers.

**14**

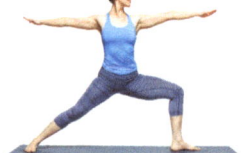

### Virabhadrasana II

-Ground the left foot between the hands.
-Pivot the right foot down and lift up.
-Stack shoulders over hips. Lift the heart.
-Lift pelvic floor.

**15**

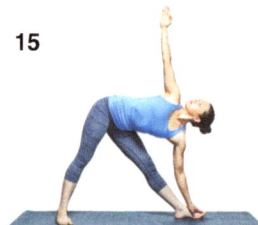

### Trikonasana

-Straighten the left leg.
-Pull the left hip back.
-Extend the side body.
-Reach forward. Release the left hand to your shin or block.
-Extend right arm up.

**16**

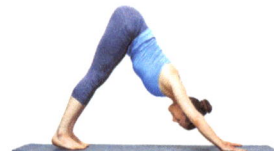

### Adho Mukha

-Spread fingers wide.
-Press the hips back.
-Lengthen the spine.
-Melt the heels down.
-Lift pelvic floor.
-Pull the belly inwards.

**17**

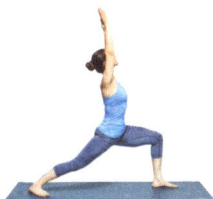

## Virabhadrasana I

-Right foot be-
tween the hands.
-Ground the edge of
the left foot down.
-Square the hips.
-Lift your arms up.
-Soften your ribs in.

**18**

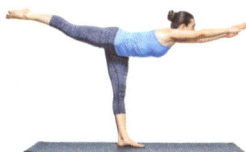

## Virabhadrasana III

-Ground into the left
foot as you lift the
right leg up behind
you, keeping hips
square to the front.
-Straight right leg.
-Reach arms forward.

**19**

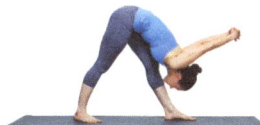

## Parsvottanasana

-Shorten your stance.
-Straighten both legs.
-Pull left hip back.
-Micro-bend left knee.
-Fold over your leg.
-Hands on floor or
blocks. Pull abs in.

**20**

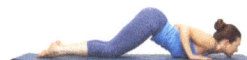

## Chaturanga

-Stack shoulders over
wrists. Lower knees to
the mat. Look forward.
-Squeeze elbows
into the ribcage as
you lower down.
-Keep shoulders back.

**21**

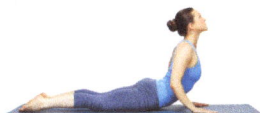

## Bhujangasana

-Place hands by chest.
-Lift the heart forward
and through the arms.
-Press into the tops of
the feet. Active legs.
-Roll shoulders back
and down the spine.

**22**

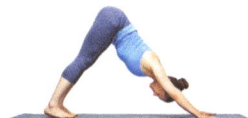

## Adho Mukha

-Spread fingers wide.
-Press the hips back.
-Lengthen the spine.
-Melt the heels down.
-Lift pelvic floor.
-Pull the belly inwards.

**23**

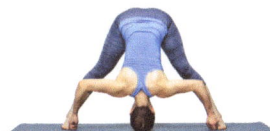

## Prasarita
## Padottanasana

-Grab your big toes.
-Fold forward in
between your legs.
-Engage the legs.
-Lengthen the spine.
-Use the abs to fold.

**24**

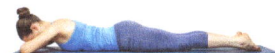

## Prone Shavasana

-Lower your fore-
head to rest on the
tops of your hands.
-Allow your entire
body to soften and
melt into the mat.
-Breathe with sound.

# Yoga Flow to BALANCE KAPHA

**1**

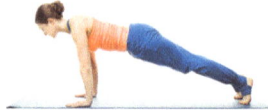

## Plank

-Bring shoulders over wrists. Lift the pelvic floor. Engage abs.
-Lengthen your low back. Broaden across the shoulders.
-Gaze soft.

**2**

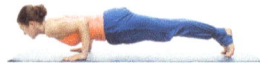

## Chaturanga

-Shift forward on your toes. Stack shoulders over wrists.
-Squeeze elbows in to the ribcage as you lower down in one line.
-Keep shoulders back.

**3**

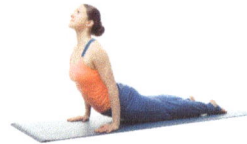

## Urdhva Mukha

-Lift the heart forward and through the arms.
-Press into the tops of the feet. Lift the legs.
-Roll shoulders back and down the spine.
-Micro-bend the arms.

**4**

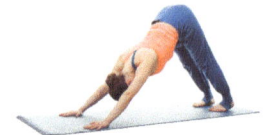

## Adho Mukha

-Spread fingers wide.
-Press the hips back as push out of the arms.
-Lengthen the spine.
-Melt the heels down.
-Lift pelvic floor.
-Pull the belly inwards.

**5**

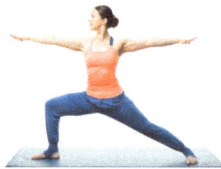

## Virabhadrasana II

-Ground the right foot between the hands.
-Pivot the left foot down and lift up.
-Stack shoulders over hips. Lift the heart.
-Pelvic floor lift.

**6**

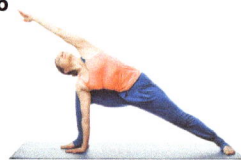

## Parsvakonasana

-Right knee over right ankle. Draw the left arm over the left ear.
-Roll right hip under.
-Stretch from the outer edge of the left foot up through the fingers.

**7**

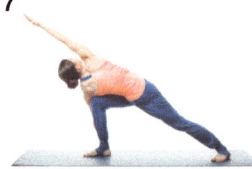

## Parivrtta Parsva-konasana

-Bring your left elbow to the outside of your right knee.
-Every inhale lengthen the spine. Exhale twist.
-Press left leg straight.

**8**

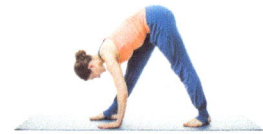

## Parsvottanasana

-Shorten your stance.
-Straighten both legs.
-Pull left hip back.
-Micro-bend left knee.
-Fold over your left leg.
-Hands on floor or blocks. Pull abs in.

Hold each pose for 3-5 deep, slow, even breaths with sound in and out the nose, creating a wave like sound with your breathing by constricting the back of the throat. Repeat the flow with the left leg and then relax in Shavasana for 5-10 minutes.

**9**

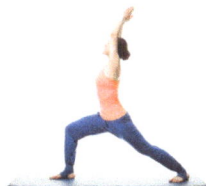

### Virabhadrasana I

-Ground the right foot between the hands.
-Square the hips forward. Ground the edge of the left foot down.
-Lift your arms up.
-Soften your ribs in.

**10**

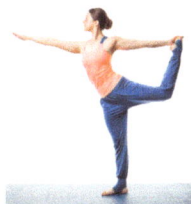

### Natarajasana

-Ground down into the right foot.
-Bend the left knee. Grab the inside edge of the left foot.
-Square hips to front.
-Kick foot into hand.

**11**

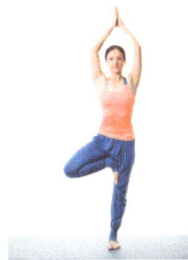

### Vrksasana

-Ground down into the left foot.
-Press the right foot to the inner thigh.
-Lift the arms, the heart. Relax shoulders.
-Engage pelvic floor.

**12**

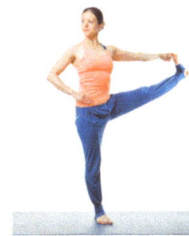

### Utthita Hasta Padangustasana

-Ground down into the right foot.
-Grab the big left toe.
-Extend the leg out to the side.
-Level the hips.

**13**

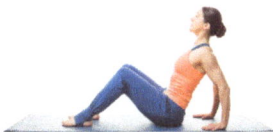

### Prep Ardha Purvottanasana

-Ground sitting bones down. Lift the heart.
-Press your feet into the floor. Long spine, engage abs, lift chest. Shoulders down.

**14**

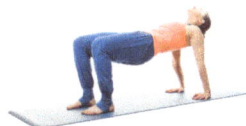

### Ardha Purvottanasana

-Fingers pointing to heels. Spread fingers.
-Press your feet into the floor and lift your seat up to knee level.
-Open across the chest.

**15**

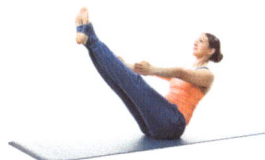

### Navasana

-Balance on sitting bones and lift legs.
-Hug legs together.
-Lengthen spine, engage core, lift chest.
-Draw shoulder blades on your back.

**16**

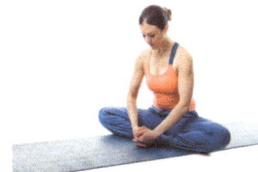

### Baddha Konasana

-Bring the soles of the feet together.
-Open feet like a book
-Extend the spine.
-Press your knees down as your fold forward with a long spine.

**17**

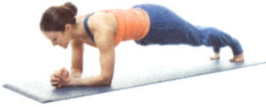

### Forearm Plank

-Hold plank pose for 10 deep, slow breaths.
-Engage your abs.
-Lengthen your tailbone towards your heels.

**18**

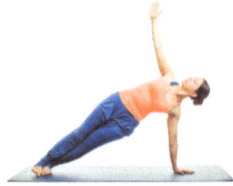

### Side Plank

-Roll over onto your forearm. Stack your feet. Lift your hips away from the floor.
-Lift he pelvic floor. Pull the navel in.
-Repeat on other side.

**19**

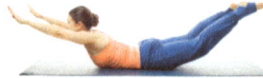

### Salabhasana

-Press the hips into the mat. Lift your arms and legs up. Length-en and lift higher.
-Squeeze inner thighs into mid line.
-Shoulders on back.

**20**

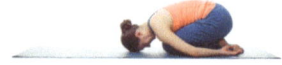

### Balasana

-Bring your feet together, open your knees, hips to heels, melt your fore-head to the floor.
-Allow the back body to soften. Breathe.

**21**

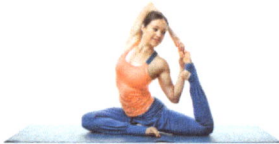

### Eka Pada Rajakapotasana

-Bend right knee in.
-Square the hips.
-Bend the left leg. Reach up and back with the right fingers for the left toes.

**22**

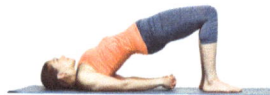

### Setu Bandha Sarvangasana

-Bring feet to the mat.
-Roll shoulders un-der. Clasp hands.
-Press into the feet. Pull inner thighs to mid line. Lift the hips

**23**

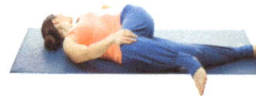

### Supta Matsyendrasana

-Lift the hips. Shift hips to right.
-Bend left knee and take it across the body.
-Stretch arms out.
-Look at left hand.

**24**

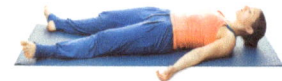

### Shavasana

-Straighten both legs.
-Roll onto your back. You can place a bol-ster under your knees.
-Pull the shoulder blades on your back.
-Relax everything.

# Weekends

## WEEKEND MORNING

Creating a habit stack for weekend mornings enables you to flow through wellness enhancing experiences before lunchtime and fills you with tranquility, energy, and joy. After drinking half a liter of water with freshly squeezed lemon, get a positive start to your day with movement. Roll right out of bed and onto your yoga mat, or head out into nature for a walk or run.

Even five minutes of movement when you first wake up will change how you feel in your body for the rest of the day. Follow movement with a more extended meditation than what you do during the week. Give yourself more time to sense your inner spaciousness and connect with joy.

Next, find a spot to curl up and read something uplifting or fascinating. The final step is to take out a journal to write in and your agenda. Analyze your past week. Review your life values. Prioritize what you want to accomplish in the next week and schedule time accordingly.

## ADVENTURE

A routine during the week filled with wellness-enhancing habits and activities is one of the best ways to feel charged with energy, balance, and contentment. A routine is also the best way to get radical progress done at work and home.

The weekend and holidays are the perfect opportunities to break free from daily life and add a kick of change and the unexpected. Permit yourself to release all the labels you've attached to your personality.

Are you sensitive to loud noise? Try going to a concert and sitting in the front.

Do you think you are the sort of person who is happiest at home with a riveting book? Go out and meet some new people in a dance class. The level of novelty, adrenaline, and surprise needed to optimize well-being differs from person to person.

Some people thrive best when they can go on a new adventure every weekend, while others only need one every few weeks. When I say adventure, I don't just mean heading out into the

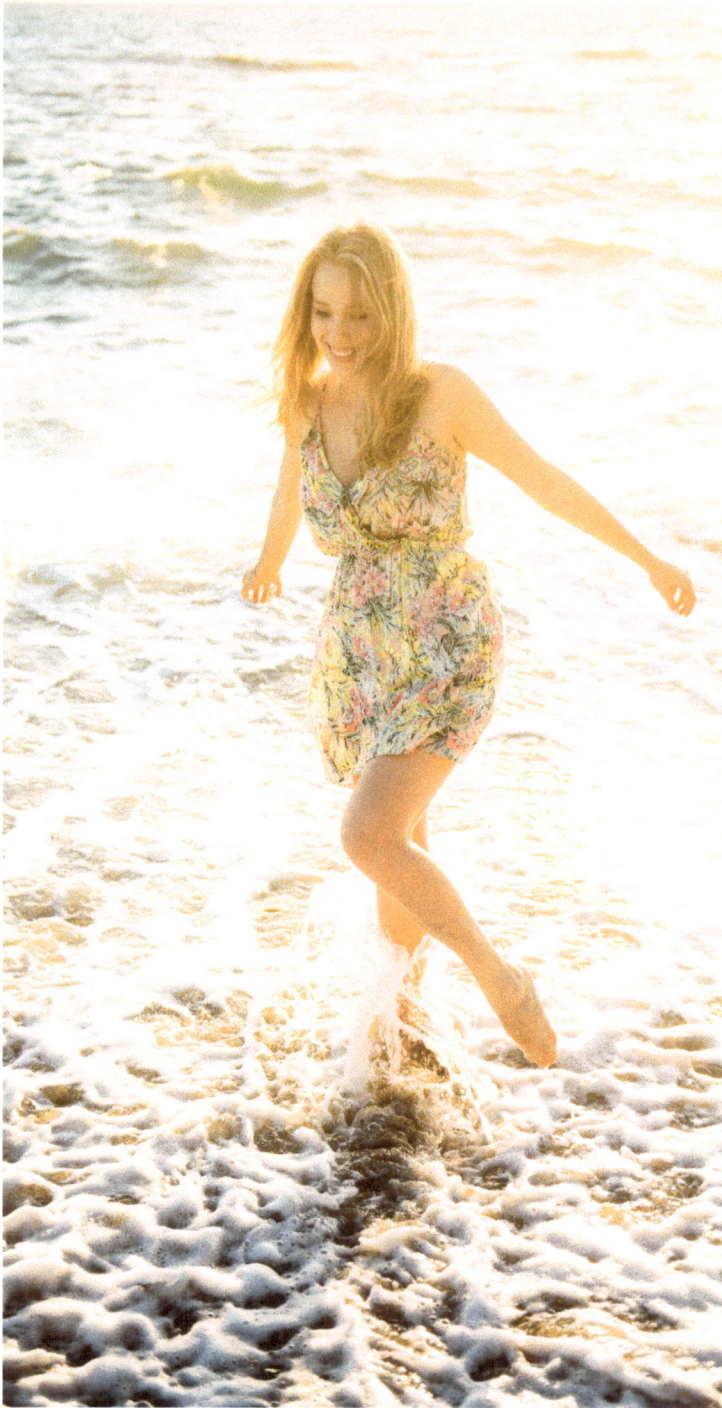

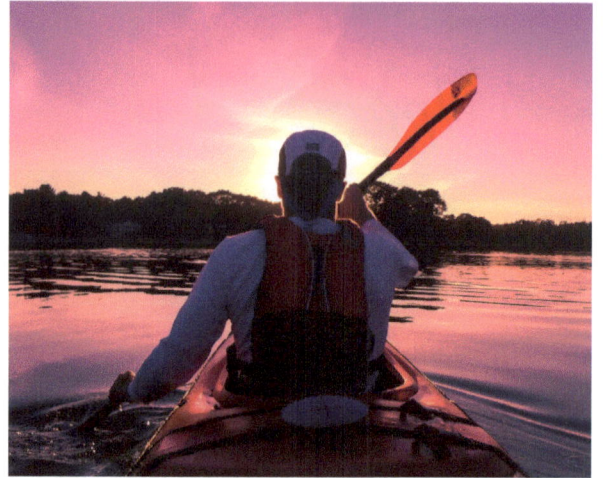

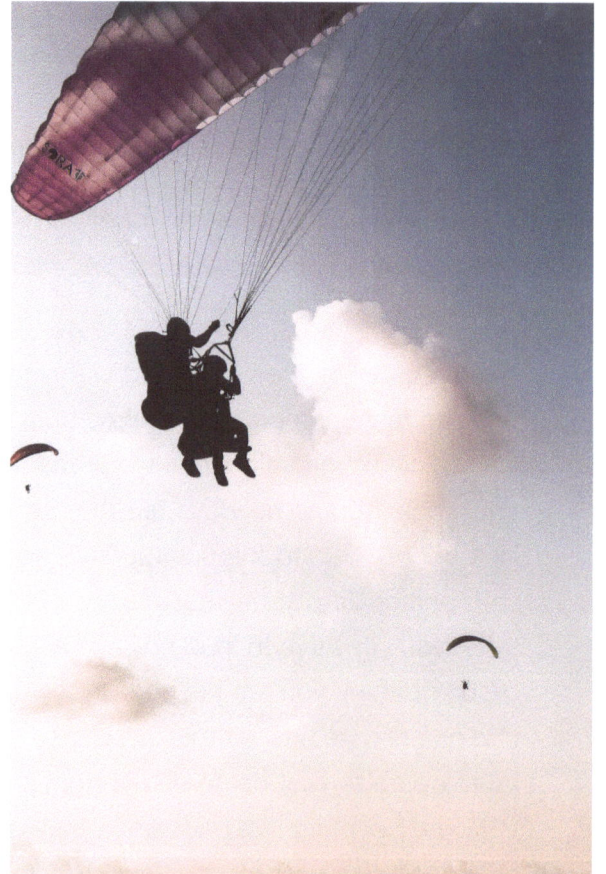

154

wilderness. Anything new or outside your comfort zone will stimulate you and anchor into your memory bank. Your adventure could be signing up for a new course, such as a cooking or photography class, going on a new hike, putting on ice-skates for the first time in your life, trying out a new fitness class, meeting new people, or traveling somewhere you've never been before for the weekend. If you are always the life of the party and never spend time alone, then your adventure could be a meditation retreat.

## REFLECTION, JOURNALING, PLANNING

*What conscious and unconscious beliefs in my physical wellness are holding me back from radiant well-being, success, and joy?*

Reflect on the different dimensions of your wellness: love, social, mental, intellectual, physical, emotional, spiritual, home, financial, work and purpose. Where are you thriving and experiencing success? In which areas of your wellness do you need to give more reflection, attention, energy, and time to elevating? We tend to view success only in terms of financial abundance and status in society or in a career. But you can experience abundance and success in
other areas such as love, physical fitness, nutrition, and self-care, or spirituality. Once you rank your success in the different areas of wellness on the next page, then set aside time to reflect and journal. What does your ideal vision for each area of your life look like? Cultivate an inner awareness as to why your vision is important to you. Know your why and values.

   What actions do you need to take to make your vision real? If you don't know, then you can search for someone who has success in this area and study the steps they took to get to where they are today.

   Consider how much time you allocate to each of the areas of wellness currently. There are only so many hours in the week.  How do you need to alter your time and energy allocation to make your visions a reality, ignite radiant wellness, and open you to more joy?

## PHYSICAL WELLNESS

Health, exercise, diet, cooking, rest, self-care

Reflect on how you feel in your body. Do you take time to move, strengthen, and stretch your body? Do you eat fresh, colorful, natural foods? Do you drink enough pure water?
Do you get eight hours of sleep a night? How well do you manage stress? Do you listen to your body and respond to its needs for movement, rest, relaxation, excitement, food, and drink?

   Do you feel good in your body? Do you feel attractive? Do you get the ideal amount and type of exercise and nutrition for your dosha type? Do you take time for self-care to feel confident and vibrant?

1. Set a vision for your ideal physical wellness.
2. Why do you want this vision of physical wellness? 3. What will you gain? What is your strategy for making your physical wellness vision a reality?
4. What actions do you need to take? How much time will these actions take?
5. Schedule the time into your ignite wellness planer.

## MENTAL WELLNESS

Meditation, sleep, diet, routine, time in nature, rest, hobbies, creativity, connection, silence

Do you get enough sleep and find time to restore after work stress and striving? Do you meditate daily? Do you eat and sleep regularly?
Do you schedule in time for beloved hobbies, creativity, time in nature, or new experiences, or do you fall into a pattern of over-work or watching TV every night?

1. Set a vision for your ideal mental wellness.
2. Why do you want this vision of mental wellness?
3. What will you gain? What is your strategy for making your mental wellness vision a reality?
4. What actions do you need to take? How much time will these actions take?

## INTELLECTUAL WELLNESS

Learning, creating, new stimulating experiences, personal development

Are you seeking out ways to continually grow and evolve as a person through personal development, learning new skills or abilities, trying new activities, or meeting new people? Are you pursuing learning to grow and stimulate your mind continually? Do you take time each day to exercise your mind?

1. Set a vision for your ideal intellectual wellness.
2. Why do you want this vision of intellectual wellness?
3. What will you gain? What is your strategy for making your intellectual wellness vision a reality?
4. What actions do you need to take? How much time will these actions take?
5. Schedule the time into your ignite wellness planer.

## EMOTIONAL WELLNESS

Loving, forgiving, connection, balance, serenity, self-love, confidence, resilience, joy

How resilient are you to stress and unfortunate events? How quickly can you forgive, yourself and others?

How well can you be in the present moment? Did you stay in touch with how you were feeling and take action to regain balance when needed? How well do you manage stress? Do you feel an inner sense of self-worth and love, feeling neither below, nor above anyone else? How often do you laugh and feel joy in daily life? How much inner balance, stillness, contentment, and serenity do you experience most of the time? Can you pause between an emotional trigger and your response?

1. Set a vision for your ideal emotional wellness.
2. Why do you want this vision of emotional wellness? 3. What will you gain? What is your strategy for making your emotional wellness vision a reality?

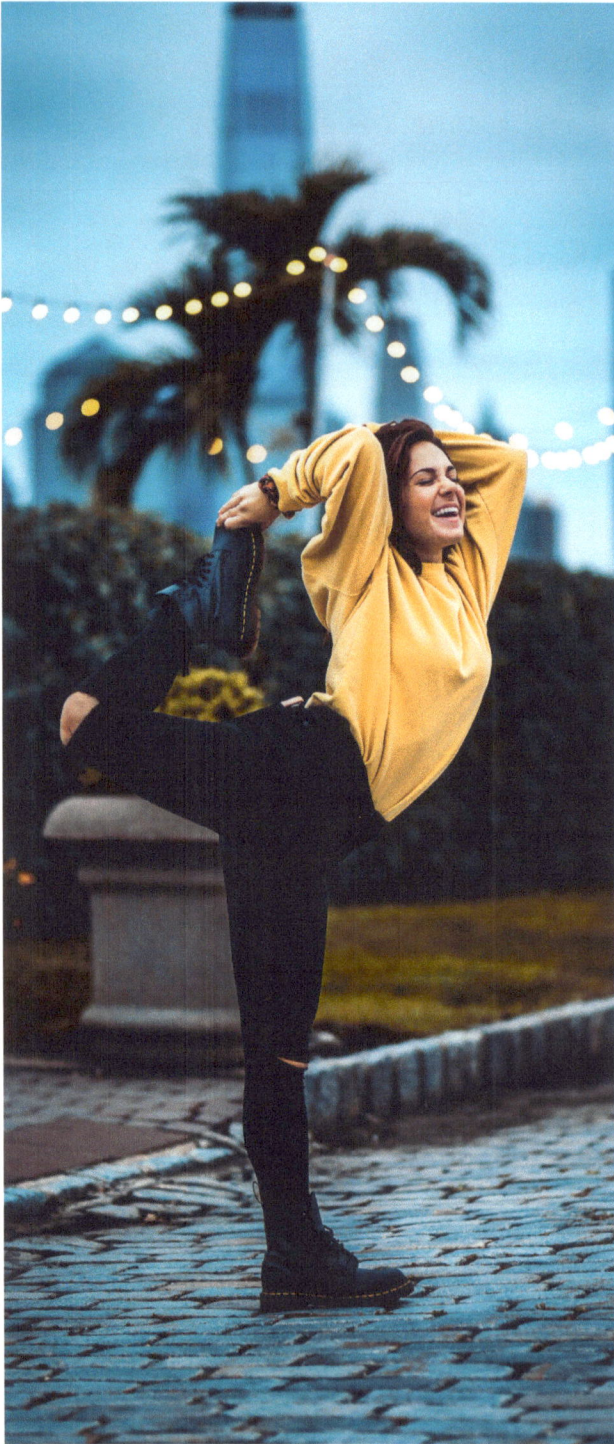
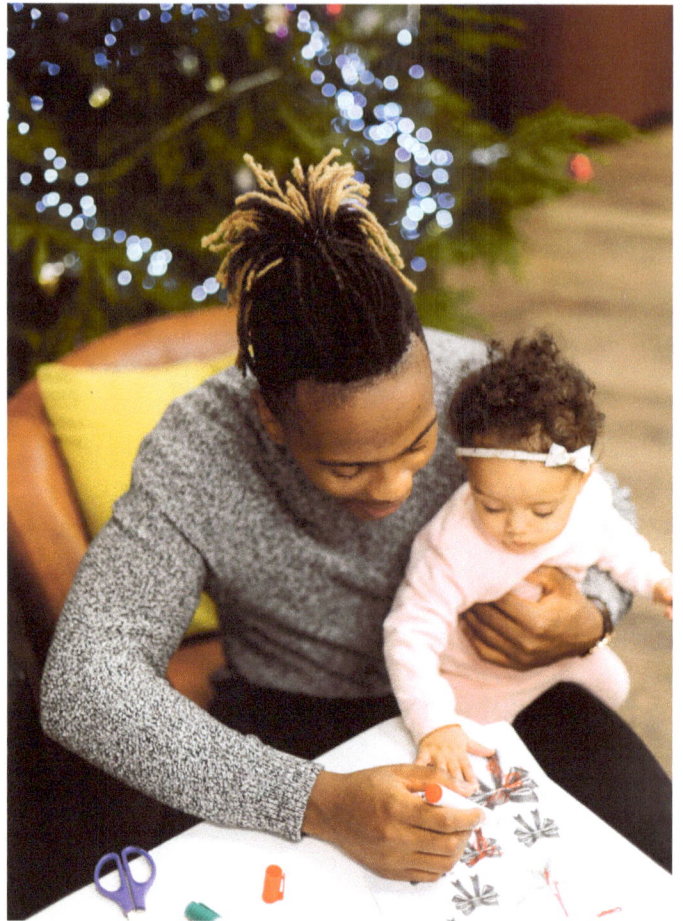
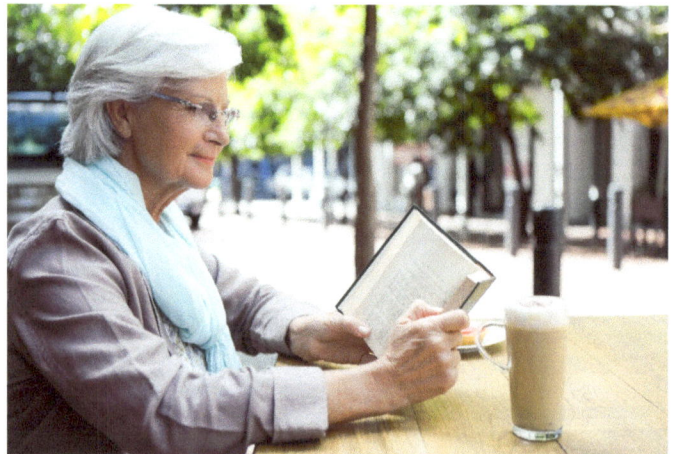

158

4. What actions do you need to take? How much time will these actions take?

5. Schedule the time into your ignite wellness planer.

## SOCIAL & LOVE WELLNESS

**Family, partner, children, friends, meeting new people, feeling part of a community**

How full of love does your life feel? How do you feel about the quality of the relationships in your life? Do you spend enough time with your loved ones? Do you need to spend more time getting out of your comfort zone and meeting new people? Are you a person of character and integrity? Do you know yourself? How well do you love? Do you engage in loving kindness? Do you spend enough time with the people who matter to you most?

Do you give the majority of your time to people that boost your energy? Do you show up as the person you want to be in each relationship? Does your life feel full of love?

1. Set a vision for your ideal social wellness.

2. Why do you want this vision of social wellness?

3. What will you gain? What is your strategy for making your social wellness vision a reality?

4. What actions do you need to take? How much time will these actions take?

5. Schedule the time into your ignite wellness planer.

## WORK & FINANCIAL WELLNESS

**Homemaking, care-giving, job, engagement for others, a sense of purpose and contribution, money, pursuing new opportunities**

Do you find purpose in your work or enjoy what you do? Is your job in alignment with your natural born constitution, leveraging your personality strengths and temperament? Do you feel that the amount of money you earn is adequate? Do you manage your finances well? Do you feel a sense of purpose? Do you feel you are contributing and making the world better? How do you feel during your work days? Are you incorporating well-being enhancing activities and behavior into your work life? Write down the progress you would like to make on medium and long-term projects for each workday for the upcoming week. Reflect on your work. Is it fulfilling? Do you feel you have found your purpose?  If not, envision what steps can you take to nourish your soul and feel fulfilled with the work, volunteer work, or free time activities.

1. Set a vision for your ideal work, homemaking, care-giving, and financial wellness.

2. Why do you want this vision of these dimensions of wellness?

3. What will you gain? What is your strategy for making your vision a reality?

4. What actions do you need to take? How much time will these actions take? Schedule the time into your ignite wellness planer.

## HOME & ENVIRONMENT WELLNESS

### Cleaning, organizing, gardening

How do you feel when you walk into your home? Were you able to create the home atmosphere you wanted? Is your home a haven and source of positive energy? Does your home ignite joy and support your sense of well-being?

   Do you garden? What about your work environment; how do you feel at work?

1. Set a vision for your ideal home, work space, garden, and even the places you vacation.

2. Why do you want this vision of wellness?

3. What will you gain? What is your strategy for making your vision a reality?

4. What actions do you need to take? How much time will these actions take?

5. Schedule the time into your ignite wellness planer.

## SPIRITUAL WELLNESS

### Meditation, prayer, inspirational reading, reflection, solitude

Do you take time daily and weekly for meditation, prayer, or and reflection? Do you actively seek out inspirational or uplifting reading, podcasts, or books? Do take time each week to nourish your soul? Do you engage in creativity? Did you take time to play? How much time did you spend in nature each day? How mindful, how present are you?

1. Set a vision for your spiritual wellness.
2. Why do you want this vision of wellness?
3. What will you gain? What is your strategy for making your vision a reality?
4. What actions do you need to take? How much time will these actions take?
5. Schedule the time into your ignite wellness planer.

## YOU KNOW YOUR VALUES & VISION. NEXT: PRIORITIZE. PLAN THE WEEK.

Take some time to sit down in a quiet place with your agenda, your value list, your list of medium and long-term goals, a notebook, and a pen.

Nothing will ignite your wellness and open you up to joy more than being present in the now. To do that, you need to set aside some time every weekend to plan out your week and write down your goals for each day in accordance with your value and vision for each dimension of wellness in your life. Otherwise, your mind will always be running through your to-do lists, and you may waste energy agonizing over how to spend your time. A sense of time pressure will creep up behind you, sending agitation and unease down your spine and into your body.

It will take some initial time investment to develop your authentic values, vision, why, and strategies. Yet with repetition and time you will automate your wellness and you will need less energy.Decide on your priorities for the week. Schedule in time for your most important priorities first thing in the morning when you are high in energy, and creativity.

Be realistic. Giving full attention to all areas of your life and wellness every day is not possible. Look at the total of the entire week.

Creating a vision, purpose, strategy, and time plan will allow a calm to settle into the depths of your being, even if the fridge is empty of food.

For instance, if you plan to give full energy and time to make a leap of progress on a project on Monday and Tuesday, then you know you will be too tired to make a gourmet meal for family

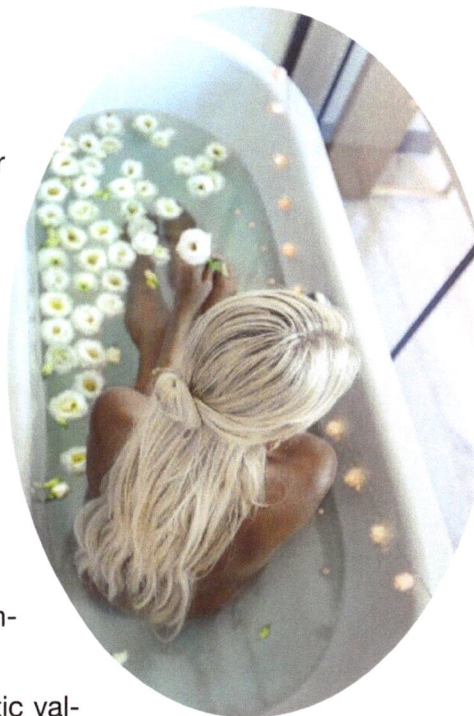

or friends in the evening and ask someone else to cook or opt for fast meals like oatmeal and berries or wholegrain pasta and pesto sauce.

## TAKE TIME TO BE GRATEFUL

Look at you analysis of the different dimensions of wellness in your life. Allow yourself to feel gratitude for the areas of your life that are thriving. Do you have loving friends? Is you social wellness wonderful? Feel thankfulness flood through your heart for everything that is abundant, beautiful, and flowing well in your life right now.

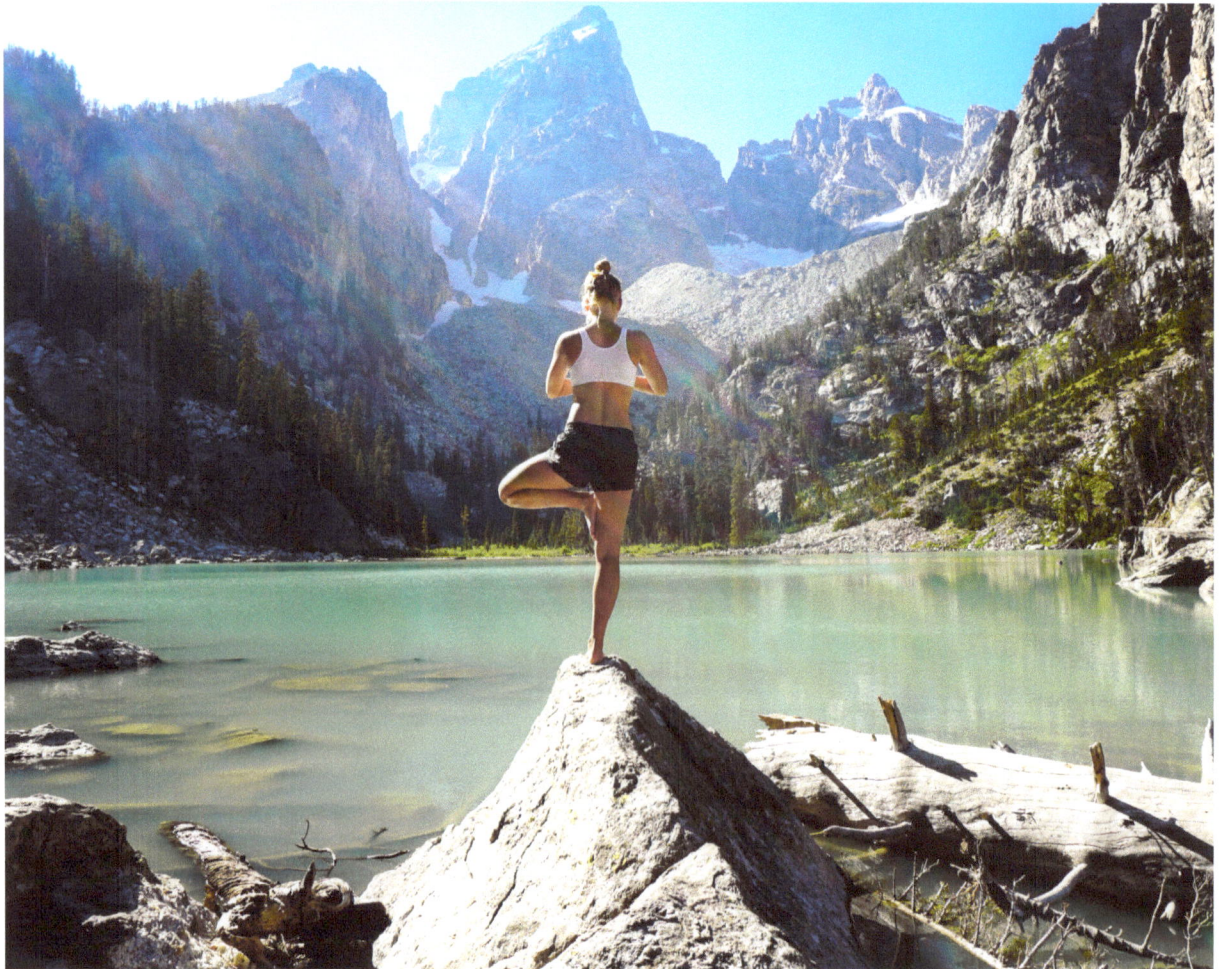

# Home Wellness Retreat

## Seeking a little serenity and renewal?

You don't need to jet to paradise to recover your glow. Press the reset button with a 4-hour wellness retreat at home.

Perhaps your job, family, or schedule keep you too busy to take a day off, let alone fly to a beach on a tropical island. This guide will enable you to seek out a few hours of wellness without leaving home or seeking out an expensive spa. Setting aside a few hours for a wellness retreat will enable you to recapture your inner and outer glow.

Once replenished, you will be better equipped to nourish those around you and work at your best.

You can even incorporate mini wellness into your everyday life with the tips and steps in this guide.

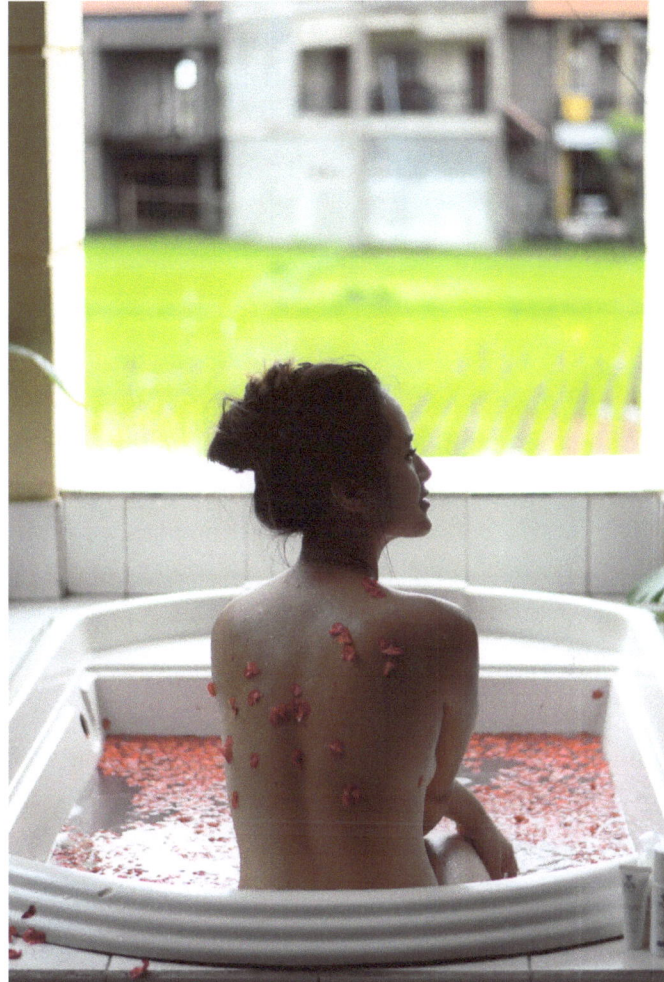

## Prepare for your home retreat.

Mark your calendar and gather the ingredients for your wellness retreat. Set a date and time for your home wellness retreat. If you have children, then find a way to carve out four hours to invest in your health and well-being. You deserve to take some time out to rejuvenate, so you can return to your life revitalized and glowing. For meals you will need ORGANIC: olive oil, vinegar, tea, 1 lemon, fresh peppermint, honey, wholegrain oatmeal, almonds, fresh or frozen blueberries, strawberries, raspberries, 1 avocado, 1 cucumber, 1 red pepper, 1 tomato, 1 can of chickpeas.

You will also need natural spa products. Treat yourself to luxurious natural, organic skin, bath, and body products for your home retreat. Short on cash? No problem. Go to the store and search for these inexpensive natural ingredients: lavender and orange essential oil, sugar, sweet almond oil, Epsom salts, a candle, paper, a pen, and 3-5 gift cards (or make your own cards.)

## Step 1. Squeeze an entire lemon into a half liter glass of water. Enjoy!

**Benefits: boosts the immune system, aids in digestion, detoxes the body, and improves skin radiance.**

One lemon contains over 100% of your daily recommended servings of vitamin C. Vitamin C boosts your immune system by stimulating white blood cell production, while the antioxidants fight free radicals in your body, rejuvenating your skin and increasing the production of collagen.

The atomic makeup of lemon juice is like your stomach's digestive juices, which signals your liver to produce bile. This helps keep food moving through your gastrointestinal tract smoothly. Lemon juice stimulates the liver to flush out more toxins while enabling you to get more nutrients out of the food you eat.

In addition to vitamin C, lemons contain vitamin B6, vitamin A, vitamin E, folate, niacin, thiamine, riboflavin, pantothenic acid, copper, calcium, iron, magnesium, potassium, zinc, and phosphorus. With so much nourishing goodness inside, it's no wonder lemons give you a radiant glow, increase your energy, and can even help you lose weight. Enjoy a glass of lemon water every day to improve digestion, immune function, and glow.

## Step 2. Enjoy a one hour vinyasa yoga session

**Benefits: enhanced well-being, stress relief, improved brain function, increased flexibility, strength, and self-love.**

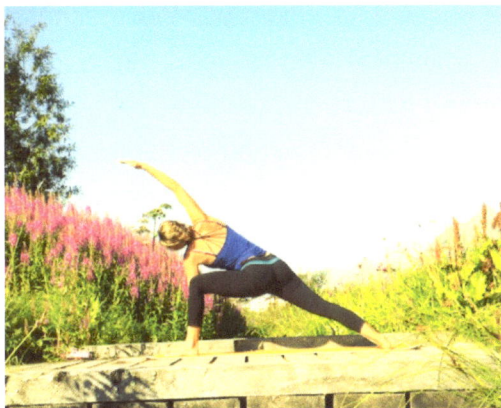
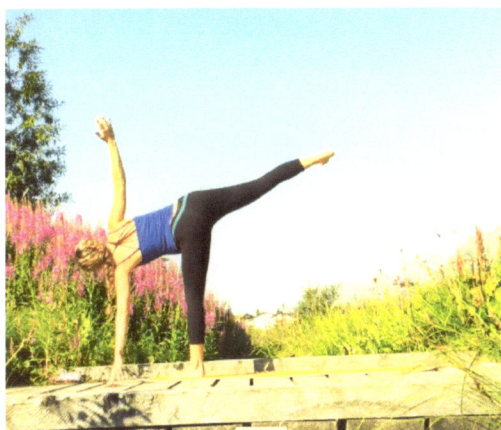
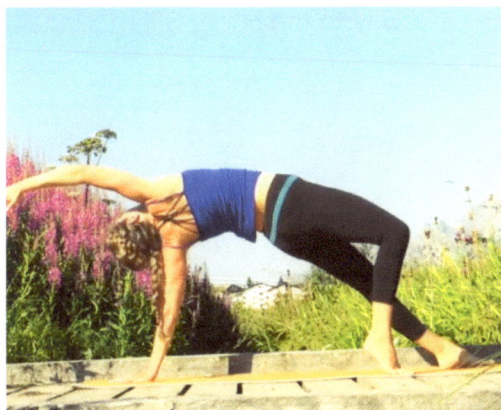
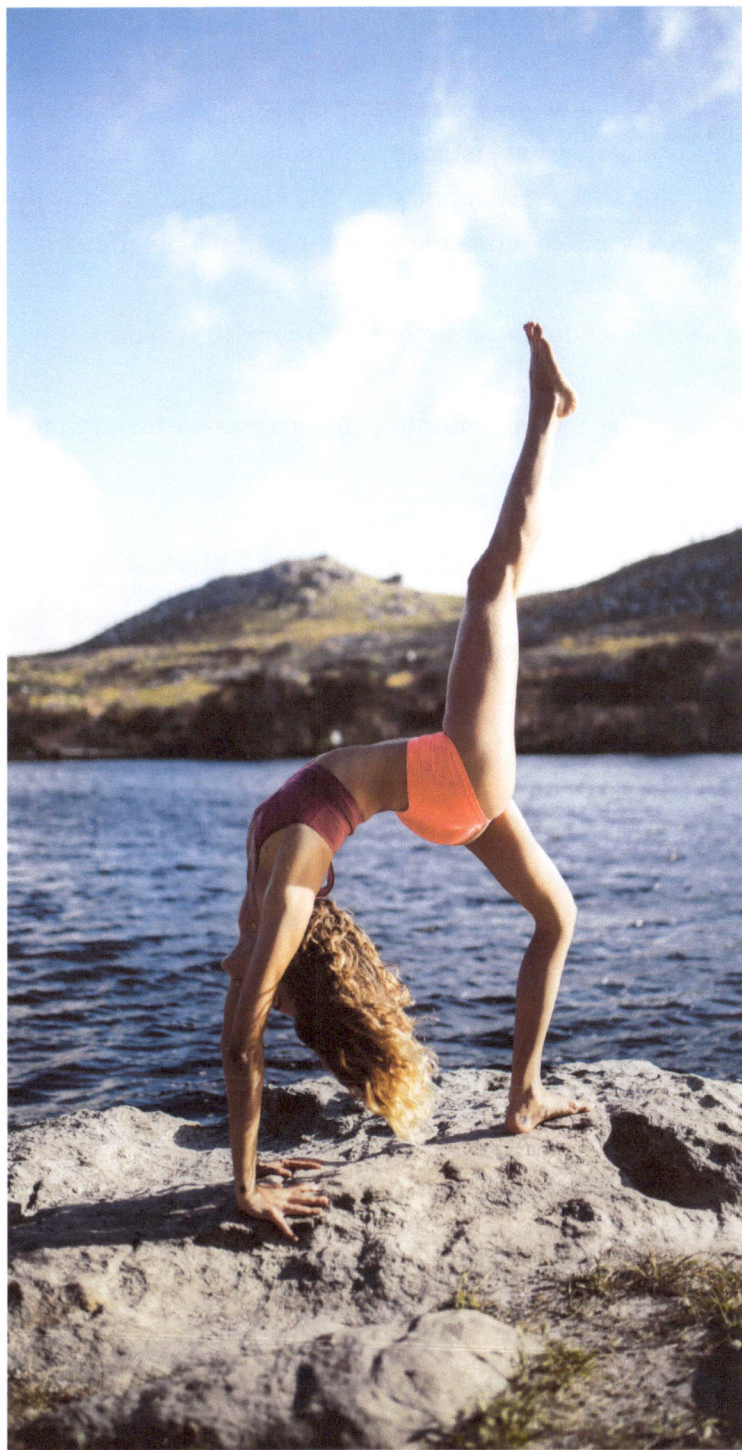

165

The benefits of yoga start from your first class. Yoga increases your inner awareness, fitness, inner peace, immunity, energy, and flexibility, and posture, while providing powerful stress relief.

Whether yoga is already a part of your life, or you are brand new to the practice, we have an hour session just for you. Practicing yoga in the cozy comfort of your own home enables you to turn inward. With no one else watching, you can try out poses you wouldn't go for in class and relax. Select one of these free classes on Youtube:

**For the Beginner Yogi: Yoga with Heather**

**For the Intermediate Yogi: Yoga with Heather Yoga Detox Vinyasa Flow to Cleanse Your Body & Energy**

**For the Advanced Yogi: Yoga with Heather Total Body**

## Step 3. Pranayama

Pranayama, or breathing exercises, increases serenity, mind - body balance, contentment, healing, and calm. Create an oasis of silence and turn your attention inward. Sit with a straight spine. Breathe in deeply through your nose. Feel your belly, front, side, and back lungs fully inflate. Breathe out slowly through your nose.

## Anxious? Stressed?

Breathe in smoothly to the count of five. Breathe out twice as slowly to the count of ten. Repeat for five minutes.

## Sluggish? Low Energy?

Start taking in short, rapid breaths through your nose in quick succession. You should feel your abs engage with each inhale. Continue for up to three minutes, then to finish take a deep breath in, hold the breath, and then exhale slowly out and come to stillness.

## Unbalanced?

Place your thumb over your right nostril. Breathe in deeply through your left nostril, then press your left nostril closed and breathe out your right nostril. Breathe in through your right nostril, then switch to breathe out your left. Repeat for 2-5 minutes.

## Step 4. Meditate & Hydrate

Rehydrate with a large glass of water with lemon juice and peppermint or cucumbers. It's time to mediate for 20 minutes. This time, find a comfortable position sitting with a tall spine. Focus on the mantra, just internally, of So Hum. Every inhalation mentally say SO, every exhale HUM. Or you can listen to one of my guided meditations on Yoga with Heather on Youtube to balance your chakras, release negativity, enter deep relaxation, or uplift your mood.

*"The process of surrender gets you to the point that you can hang loose, without the urge to grab at things and worry over them... your mind learns what it's like to be quiet, comfortable and loose." - Deepak Chopra*

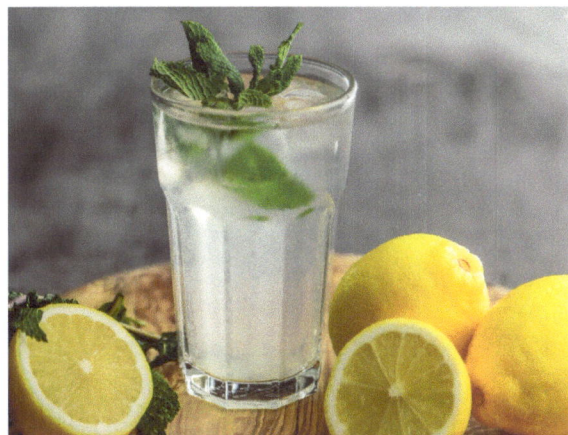

## Step 5. Enjoy a Yin Yoga Class and Yoga Nidra to Replenish and Release

Benefits: rejuvenation, enhanced well-being, stress relief, emotional release, healing, increased flexibility, deep relaxation, and self-love.

In the comfort of your own home, with no one watching, you can open up and relax. Let this Yin Yoga session bring up any stress or negative emotions that have condensed in your body. Becoming still and going inward will allow you to unlock and release emotions and find healing.

With no one else watching, you can cry, laugh out loud, or scream into a pillow. This is your time to shed anything weighing on your energy and dulling your sparkle. Let's rekindle your glow. Try one of the following free Yin Yoga classes on Yoga with Heather on Youtube and finish with the Yoga Nidra:

**For the Beginner Yogi: Yoga with Heather DETOX Yin Yoga**

**For the Intermediate Yogi: Yoga with Heather Chakra Healing Yin Yoga**

**Yoga Nidra**

## Step 6. Nourish Your Body

Prepare a bowl of whole grain oatmeal and berries. Enjoy a cup of organic tea.

Resist the urge to check social media, turn on the TV, or the news. Digitally detox yourself. Instead, enjoy the stillness or turn on the sound of ocean waves. Preparing a healthy meal doesn't need to take too much effort or time. Prepare a bowl of warm, comforting goodness.

**Directions:**

First combine 1 cup whole grain oats, 1 teaspoon of cinnamon, 1 cup of milk, 1 cup of water, a pinch of salt, and in a medium saucepan. Bring to a boil, then reduce heat to low. Next simmer uncovered for 3 to 5 minutes until thickened, stirring occasionally. Remove from heat and let

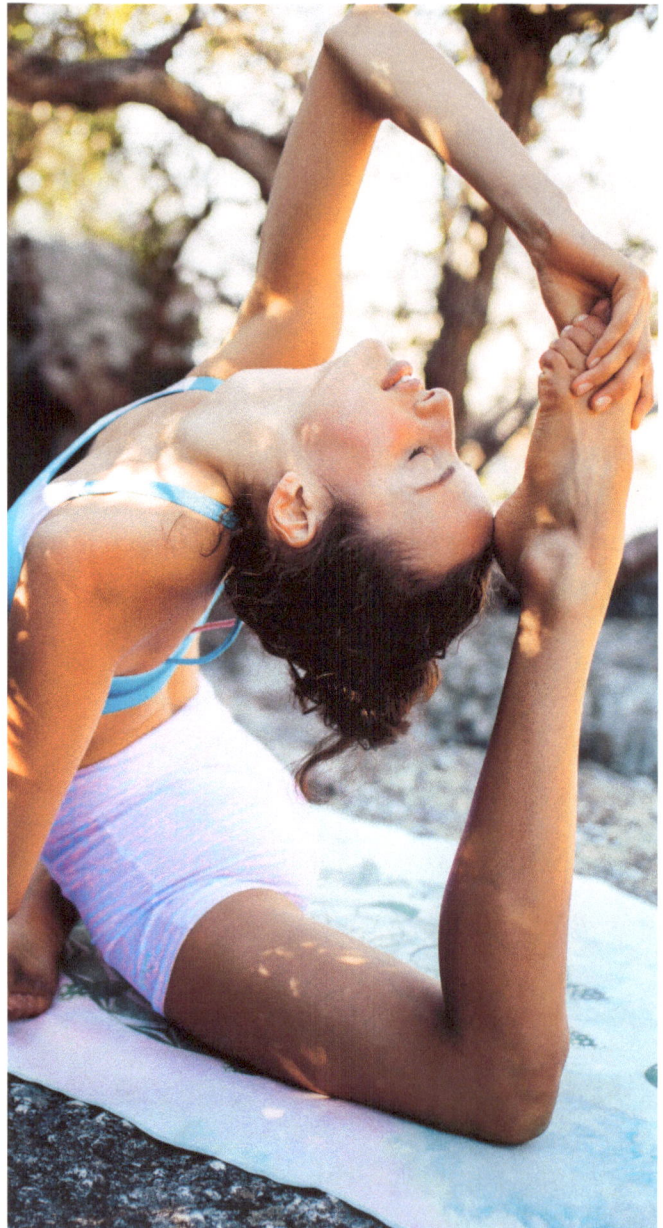

cool slightly. Last add blueberries, strawberries, and raspberries to your oatmeal; add honey to sweeten as desired. Enjoy a glass of organic tea to rehydrate.

## Step 7. Run a Bath

Benefits: Smooth skin, relaxation, open pores for skin detox, chakra balancing.

Add five tablespoons of sugar to a bowl. Squeeze in the juice from half a lemon and add one drop of essential orange oil and one tablespoon of olive oil. Run a bath and add your bath bomb or salts, or add your Epsom salts and five to ten drops of orange organic essential oil. Light your beeswax tea light to create a relaxing ambiance. Relax into the bath.

The fruity-citric fragrance should boost your mood and encourage you to feel cheerful and optimistic. Be sure your bath isn't too hot, or it will stress your body and dry out your skin. Relax in the bath for 20 minutes.

### Skin renewal.

Next, use your homemade scrub to massage your face and body in circular motions. Pay attention to rough areas on your elbows, knees, and feet. Rinse off before ending your bathing experience. Your skin should feel soft and supple.

## Step 8.  Cold Shower

Ready for an energy kick and to kick your immune system into high gear? Turn the water to icy cold. Place your right leg under the cold water and count to thirty. Switch legs. Next, place your right arm under the cold water to the shoulder and count to thirty. Switch arms. Now, how brave are you? Jump in and let the water run over your face. Turn and feel the cold rush down along your spine while counting to sixty.

The cold water rush provides a natural shock to your body causing oxygen intake to increase as well as your heart rate. Blood circulation is improved as the cold water hits your skin. This will leave you feeling invigorated after your shower and full of energy. Daily cold showers can also improve your muscle recovery after workouts, strengthen your immune system, reduce stress, help depression and lead to easier weight loss. A daily cold water plunge even increases our levels of willpower and self-control; it gives us an energy kick that lasts for hours.

## Step 9. Skin care, Self care

**Benefits:** deeply relaxing and hydrating, smooths the skin, granting it a smooth texture and natural glow.

Get your organic olive or sweet almond oil. Natural oils are the perfect moisture and nutrient dispenser with a fine texture that is completely absorbed into the skin. The daily massaging of the natural oil into the skin improves blood circulation, hydrates, and supports the skins ability to serve as a healthy barrier to toxins and bacteria. You should apply the body oil right after the shower when your skin is still a little wet. Start with a few drops to your palm with one drop of essential lavender oil.

Massage the oil in long smooth strokes down the muscles in your arms and legs. Massage the oil in a clockwise, circular motion first to your stomach and back, then on each joint: wrists, elbows, shoulders, hips, knees, and ankles. Finish by massaging the oil into your feet. This Ayurveda massage is deeply relaxing; it will calm your nerves, lubricate your joints and improve your skin, energy levels, and sleep.

## Step 10. Face care, Cleanse, Detox

**Benefits:** dissolves the oily impurities in your skin, melting away daily grime, black heads, while gently ex-foliating, hydrating, refreshing, anti-aging.

1. Cleanse deeply and melt away grime with an ex-foliating cleanser. Mix a drop of ex-foliating cleanser in your hands with

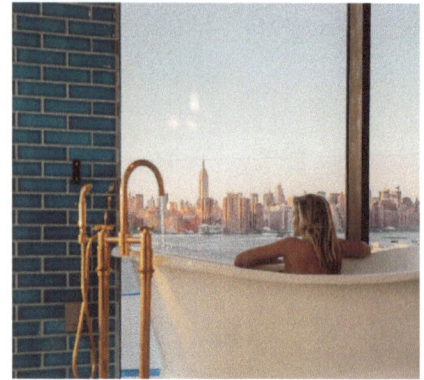

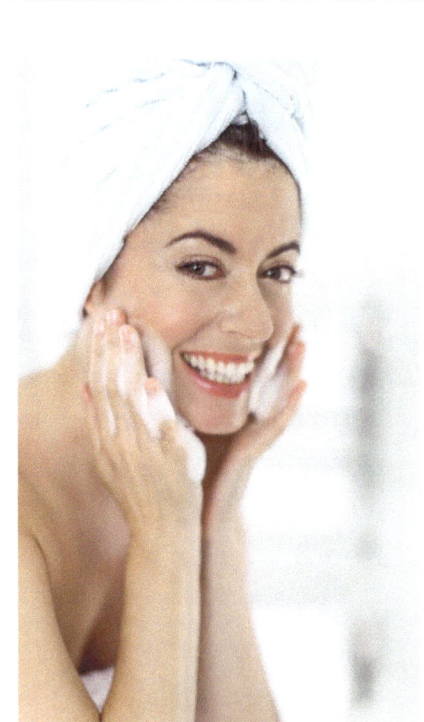

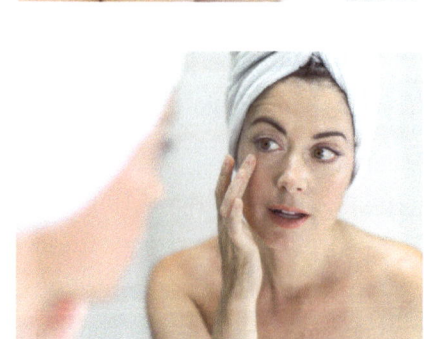

a few drops warm water. Massage into your face for two minutes and remove with warm water.

2. Detox with a mineral mask. Mix equal parts of dry mask and water (about one tsp of each). Or, you can combine a mud mask with yogurt or honey instead of water. Don't be alarmed if you get a blemish the following day - this does occasionally happen because of impurities being drawn to the skin's surface.

This is a good thing because it means the mask is doing its job. Re-apply a small amount of mask to the problem area.

3. Refresh, tone, and balance with a hydrating facial Rose water spray. Shake the bottle before use, then spray onto your face and neck until moist while holding the bottle 10-15 cm away from your face.

4. Moisturize with facial oil. Apply 1 to 5 drops to your slightly damp face and neck to give stressed- out skin a velvety smooth complexion. You can select an organic olive, sweet almond, jojoba, apricot kernel, tea tree, argan, grapefruit or avocado oil.

Select an oil based on your skin type that will work with your skin for optimal absorption and nourishment. Organic face oils provides a heavy-weight hit of nourishing goodness that feels divinely silky when applied. Facial oil can simultaneously retain moisture, reduce the chance of bacterial invasion and balance sebum production for a healthy skin barrier.

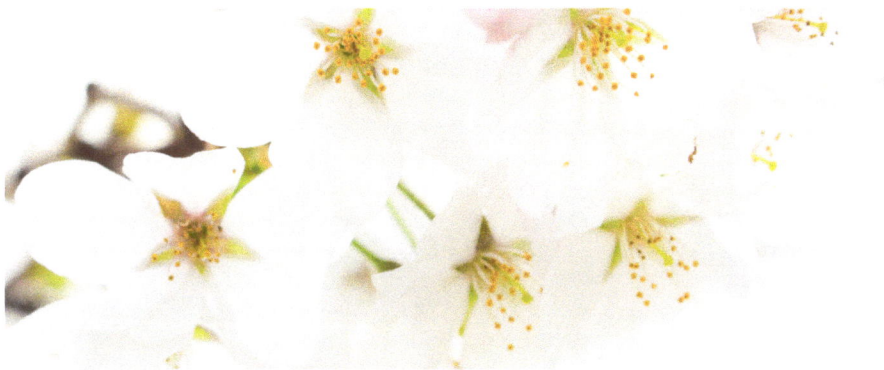

## Almond Oil

A great moisturizing oil, capable of helping to even out skin tone and reduce scars, almond oil's B vitamins and healthy fats help fight the signs of aging.

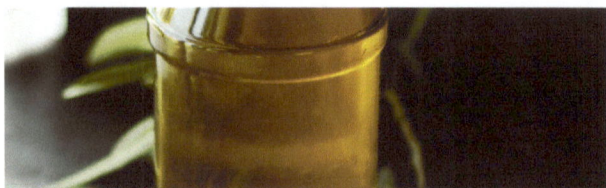

## Olive Oil

Intense moisturizer, a cleanser, and a sun-damage protector, olive oil can be applied straight to the skin and hair. Its monosaturated fatty acids fight inflammation.

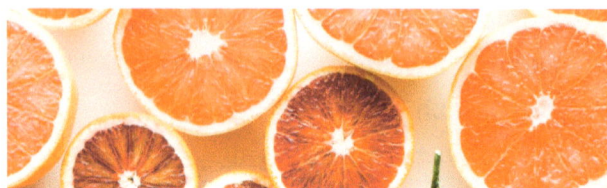

## Grapefruit Oil

Contains the enzyme bromelain, which exfoliates the uppermost layers of the skin. A serious anti-inflammatory, it aids in fighting psoriasis and acne.

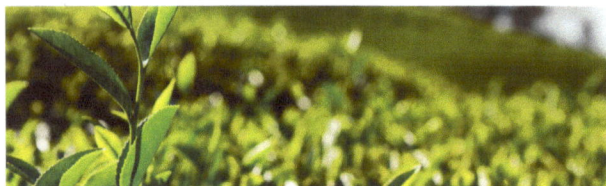

## Jojoba Seed Oil

A non-greasy, anti-inflammatory oil, jojoba oil helps moisturize the skin, without clogging the pores. It is antibacterial, oil controlling, and reduces wrinkles.

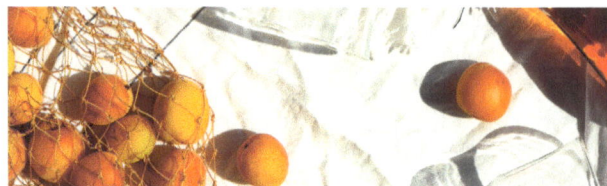

## Apricot Kernel Oil

It sinks into the skin without leaving a greasy feel behind. It contains lots of good fatty acids, vitamins A, C, and E (all skin-boosters!), and it's a gentle anti-inflammatory.

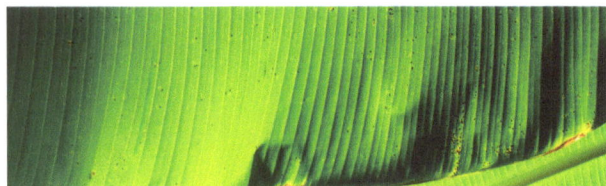

## Tea Tree Oil

A champion anti-viral and anti-fungal substance. It kills acne bacteria, heals cuts and sores faster, chases away any kind of lil' nasty microscopic critter living on you.

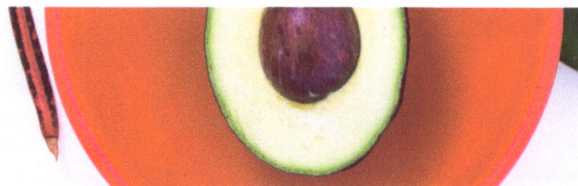

## Avocado Oil

It is a moisturizing superstar with one of the highest levels of vitamin E, making it excellent for fighting the free radicals that want to make your skin age faster.

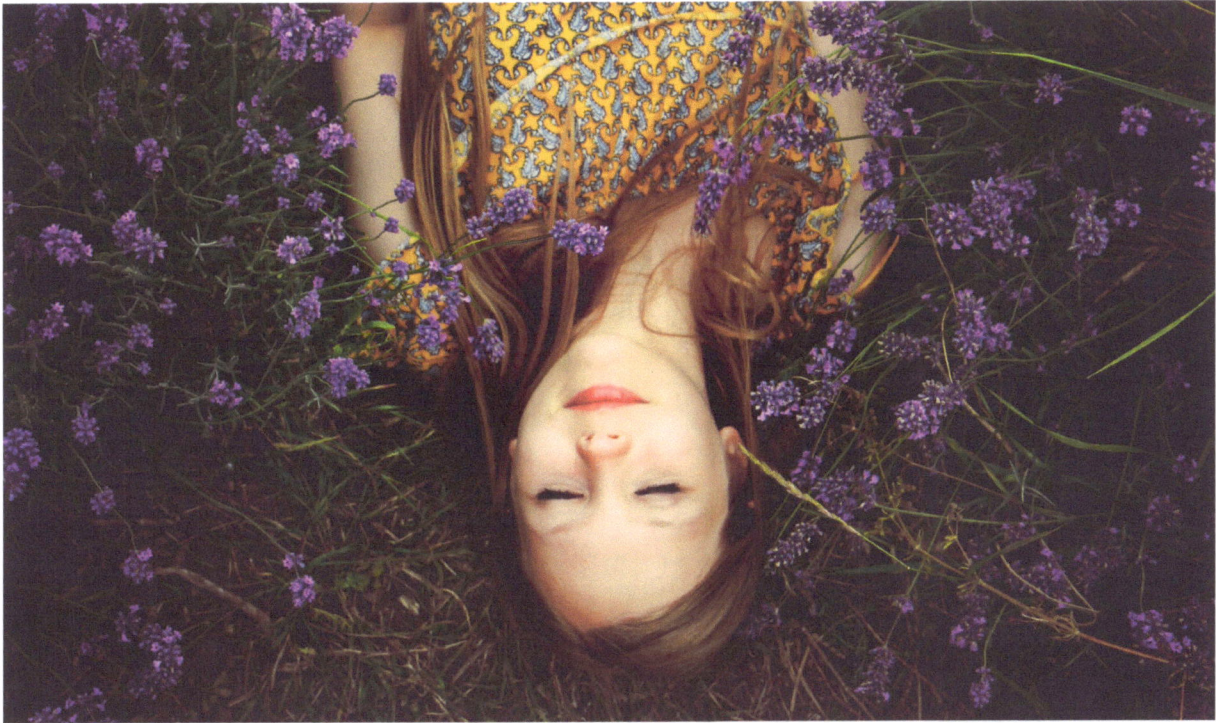

## Step 11. Nourish your body, then rest

**Prepare Your Multi-colored Salad.** Cut up one avocado, one red pepper, half a cucumber, one tomato and add one can of cooked chickpeas. Add a tablespoon of olive oil and vinegar.

You deserve a rest. Curl up in your bed or on your coach and enjoy the restorative effects of taking time out to read or take a nap.

Next, prepare a cup of tea. Take the steaming cup of tea outside to savor in the fresh air in silence. If this isn't possible, appreciate green indoor plants, flowers, or a bowl of fresh fruit.

Contemplate the beauty of nature while you let any emotions bubble up to the surface. Notice any feelings or ideas that were suppressed by daily noise, constant activity, and technology. Take your paper and pen out. Write cards to someone in your life telling them what you love most about them. Next, journal for ten minutes about at least ten things, people, or experiences for which you are grateful. Your wellness retreat is now complete.

I hope you have nourished your body, mind, and spirit and can return to your life feeling delicious and glowing with vitality.

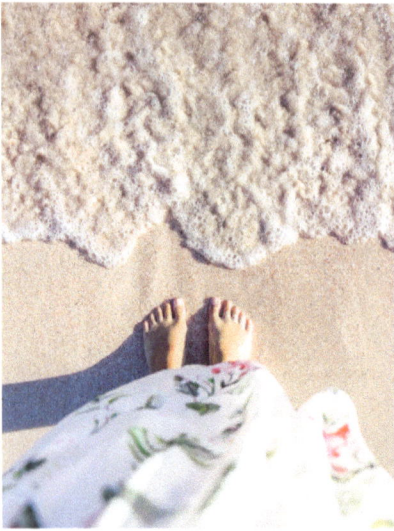

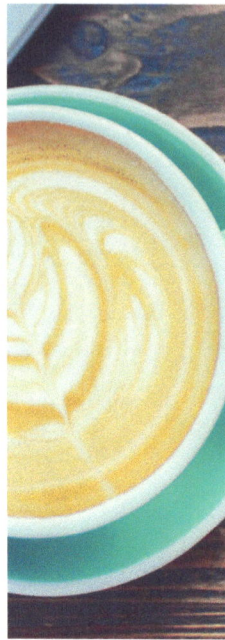

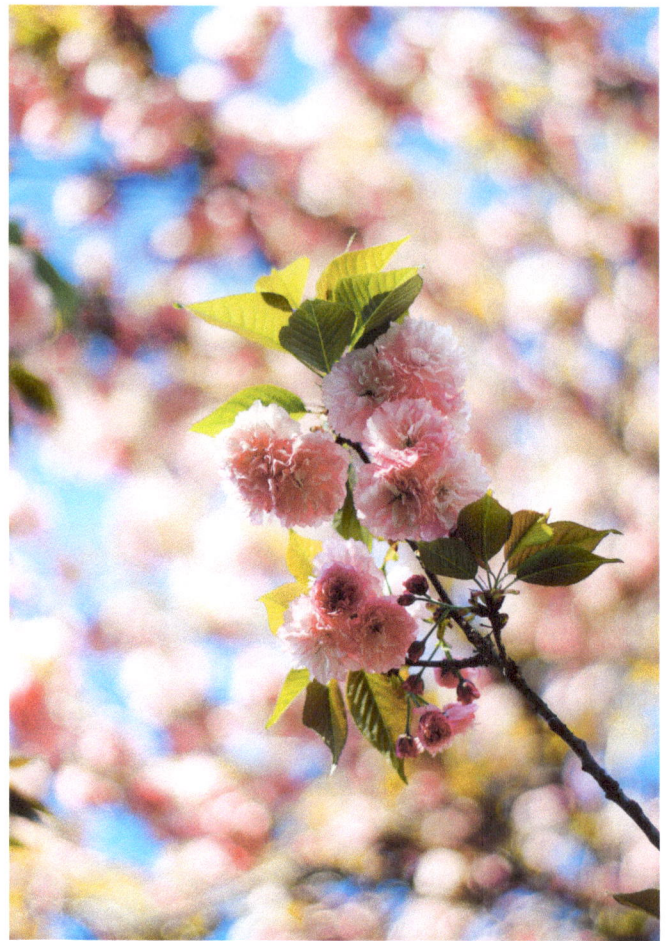

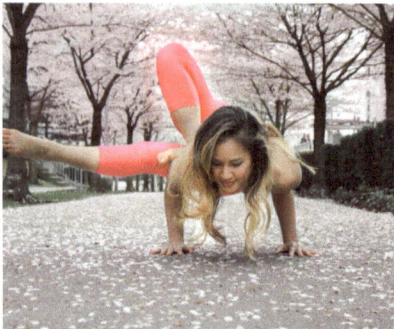

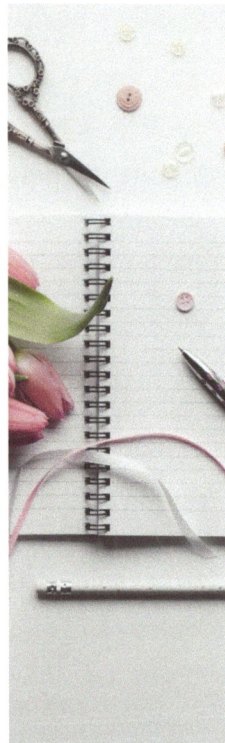

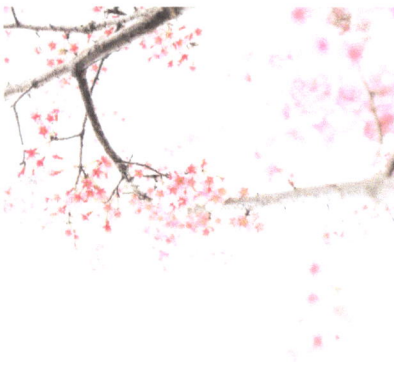

"Becoming conscious of stillness whenever we encounter it in our lives will connect us with the formless and timeless dimension within ourselves, that which is beyond thought, beyond ego. It may be the stillness that pervades the world of nature, or the stillness in your room in the early hours of the morning, or the gaps between sounds... To be still is to be conscious without thought. You are never more essentially, more deeply yourself than when you are still."
 - Eckhart Tolle

# Note from the author.

What I know for sure is we are all challenged in different ways in this lifetime. For you it could be your weight, aches and pains in your body, insomnia, addiction to drama, or something else. What we share is a desire to feel healthy and happy. I hope this book helps get you closer :)

Writing this book is a wish from the bottom of my soul to help anyone who can benefit in any small way by my journey to feeling blissful, beautiful, and balanced in body, mind, and spirit. Okay, so I don't feel like that all the time. (But it would be AMAZING, am I right?)

The essential point is that I use the steps in this book as a guide to bring myself BACK into well-being over and over again in regular daily living. You can too!

Life can throw you curve balls. People can be challenging. It's empowering to have a set of principles that empowers us to start to flow quicker and quicker back into balance in daily life, no matter what person, surprise or hardship we meet.

Are you living your life with conscious intention? Is your life filled with meaning? What sparks joy in your life? What makes your body, mind, and spirit feel blissful, beautiful, and balanced? How can you add more of this bliss into your daily routine?

I'm on a lifelong mission to make these your go-to questions. I believe when we focus on what opens us to joy, purpose, health, and wellness, instead of on our current profession, belongings, or even emotions, we rise above. We enter a place of being. WELL-being. And it's so much easier to let love flow out from a place of well-BEING.

Being in the present moment is where the magic happens. So let's dive into the expansive stillness inside, and along the way find ways to add more health, serenity, joy, purpose, and a whole lot of LOVE into daily life. It can start with this breath. Now.

Let's take this wellness journey together. Connect and share what brings you joy:

Email       adeliciousglow@gmail.com
Instagram   yogawithheathernadine
Youtube     Yoga with Heather

Wishing you radiant health, joy & so much love — Heather

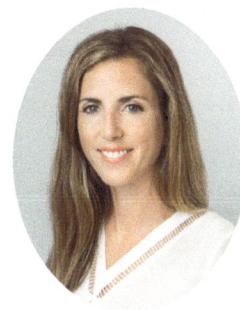

# REFERENCES

## ARTICLES

1.      Kujala UM1, Kaprio J, Sarna S, Koskenvuo M. Relationship of leisure-time physical activity and mortality: the Finnish twin cohort. JAMA. 1998 Feb 11;279(6):440-4. https://www.ncbi.nlm.nih.gov/pubmed/9466636

2.      Hamer M1, Chida Y. Walking and primary prevention: a meta-analysis of prospective cohort studies. Br J Sports Med. 2008 Apr;42(4):238-43. Epub 2007 Nov 29. https://www.ncbi.nlm.nih.gov/pubmed/18048441

3.      Walking: Your steps to health; Walking for health. Harvard University Medical School. Harvard Health Publishing. 2009. https://www.health.harvard.edu/exercise-and-fitness/walking-for-health

4.      Cheng HP, Chen CH, Lin MH, Wang CS, Yang YC,5, Lu FH, Wu JS, Lin SI. Gender differences in the relationship between walking activity and sleep disturbance among community-dwelling older adult with diabetes in Taiwan. J Women Aging. 2017 Dec 22:1-9. doi: 10.1080/08952841.2017.1413830. [Epub ahead of print] https://www.ncbi.nlm.nih.gov/pubmed/29272219

5.      Breneman CB, Kline CE, West DS, Sui X, Porter RR, Bowyer KP, Custer S, Wang. The effect of moderate-intensity exercise on nightly variability in objectively measured sleep parameters among older women. Behav Sleep Med. 2017 Oct 20:1-11. doi: 10.1080/15402002.2017.1395337. [Epub ahead of print] https://www.ncbi.nlm.nih.gov/pubmed/29053410

6.      Yuenyongchaiwat K. Effects of 10,000 steps a day on physical and mental health in overweight participants in a community setting: a preliminary study. Braz J Phys Ther. 2016 Jun 16. pii: S1413-35552016005008102. doi: 10.1590/bjpt-rbf.2014.0160. [Epub ahead of print]

7.      Samuel B. Harvey, F.R.A.N.Z.C.P., Ph.D., Simon Øverland, Ph.D., Stephani L. Hatch, Ph.D., Simon Wessely, F.R.C.Psych., M.D., Arnstein Mykletun, Ph.D., Matthew Hotopf, F.R.C.Psych., Ph.D. Exercise and the Prevention of Depression: Results of the HUNT Cohort Study. The American Journal of Psychiatry. October 03, 2017.

8.      Gregory N. Bratmana, J. Paul Hamiltonb, Kevin S. Hahnc, Gretchen C. Dailyd,e, and James J. Grossc. Social Sciences - Psychological and Cognitive Sciences: Nature experience reduces rumination and subgenual prefrontal cortex activation. PNAS 2015 112 (28) 8567-8572; published ahead of print June 29, 2015, doi:10.1073/pnas.1510459112 http://www.pnas.org/content/112/28/8567.full

9.      REBECCA A. CLAY. Green is good for you. Monitor on Psychology. April 2001, Vol 32, No. 4. Print version: page 40.

10.     Dongying Li  William C. Sullivan. Impact of views to school landscapes on recovery from stress and mental fatigue. University of Illinois, Department of Landscape Architecture. https://aslathedirt.files.wordpress.com/2016/01/li-sullivan.pdf

11.     Wells, N.M., & Evans, G. W. (2003). Nearby nature a buffer of life stress among rural children. Environment and Behavior, 35(3), 311–330.

12.     Wood L, Hooper P, Foster S, Bull F. Public green spaces and positive mental health - investigating the relationship between access, quantity and types of parks and mental wellbeing. Health Place. 2017 Nov;48:63-71. doi: 10.1016/j.healthplace.2017.09.002. Epub 2017 Sep 23.

13.     Juan Jiang, Margo P. Emont1, Heejin Jun, Xiaona Qiao, Jiling Liao, Dong-il Kim, Jun Wu'. Cinnamaldehyde induces fat cell-autonomous thermogenesis and metabolic reprogramming. December 2017Volume 77, Pages 58–64.

14.     Murray-Stewart T, Casero RA. Regulation of Polyamine Metabolism by Curcumin for Cancer Prevention and Therapy. Johns Hopkins University. Med Sci (Basel). 2017 Dec 18;5(4). pii: E38. doi: 10.3390/medsci5040038.

15.     Obaidi, Higgins, Bahar, Davis JL, McMorrow T. Identification of the multifaceted chemopreventive activity of curcumin against the carcinogenic potential of the food additive, KBrO3Curr Pharm Des. 2017 Dec 26. doi: 10.2174/1381612824666171226143201. [Epub ahead of print] Food Funct. 2015 Mar;6(3):910-9. doi: 10.1039/c4fo00680a.

16.     Gunawardena D, Karunaweera N, Lee S, van Der Kooy F, Harman DG, Raju R, Bennett L, Gyengesi E, Sucher NJ, Münch G. Anti-inflammatory activity of cinnamon (C. zeylanicum and C. cassia) extracts - identification of E-cinnamaldehyde and o-methoxy cinnamaldehyde as the most potent bioactive compounds.

17.     Pasupuleti Visweswara Rao  and Siew Hua Gan . Cinnamon: A Multifaceted Medicinal Plant. 10.2174/1381612824666171226143201.

18.     Lopresti AL. Curcumin for neuropsychiatric disorders: a review of in vitro, animal and human studies. Food Funct. 2015 Mar;6(3):910-9. doi: 10.1039/c4fo00680a. Evid Based Complement Alternat Med. 2014. J Psychopharmacol. 2017

19.     https://www.healthline.com/health/turmeric-for-skin#skin-benefits2 Turmeric for Skin: Benefits and Risks.

20.     Greger, Michael. How Not to Die. Pan Books, 2017.

21.     https://draxe.com/10-medicinal-ginger-health-benefits/

22.     Pashaei-Asl R, Pashaei-Asl F, Mostafa Gharabaghi P, Khodadadi K, Ebrahimi M, Ebrahimie E, Pashaiasl M. The Inhibitory Effect of Ginger Extract on Ovarian Cancer Cell Line; Application of Systems Biology. Ginger Health Benefits. Adv Pharm Bull. 2017 Jun;7(2):241-249. doi: 10.15171/apb.2017.029.

23.     Ozgoli G, Goli M, Moattar F. Comparison of effects of ginger, mefenamic acid, and ibuprofen on pain in women with primary dysmenorrhea. J Altern Complement Med. 2009 Feb;15(2):129-32. doi: 10.1089/acm.2008.0311.

24.     Maghbooli M, Golipour F, Moghimi Esfandabadi A, Yousefi M. Comparison between the efficacy of ginger and sumatriptan in the ablative treatment of the common migraine. Phytother Res. 2014 Mar;28(3):412-5. doi: 10.1002/ptr.4996. Epub 2013 May 9.

25.     Shoba G, Joy D, Joseph T, Majeed M, Rajendran R, Srinivas PS. Influence of piperine on the pharmacokinetics of curcumin in animals and human volunteers. Planta Med. 1998 May;64(4):353-6. Nutr Metab (Lond).

26.     Meriga, Parim, Chunduri, Naik, Nemani, Suresh, Ganapathy, Vvu. Antiobesity potential of Piperonal: promising modulation of body composition, lipid profiles and obesogenic marker expression in HFD-induced obese rats. https://www.ncbi.nlm.nih.gov/pubmed/29176994

27.     Rahman MM, Alam MN, Ulla A, Sumi FA, Subhan N, Khan T, Sikder B, Hossain H, Reza HM, Alam MA. Cardamom powder supplementation prevents obesity, improves glucose intolerance, inflammation and oxidative stress in liver of high carbohydrate high fat diet induced obese rats. 2017 Nov 16;14:72.

28.     Qiu L, Sautter J, Liu Y, Gu D. Age and gender differences in linkages of sleep with subsequent mortality and health among very old Chinese. Sleep Med. 2011 Dec;12(10):1008-17. doi: 10.1016/j.sleep.2011.04.014. Epub 2011 Oct 28. https://www.ncbi.nlm.nih.gov/pubmed/22036598

29.     Patyar S, Patyar RR. Correlation between Sleep Duration and Risk of Stroke. J Stroke Cerebrovasc Dis. 2015 May;24(5):905-11. doi: 10.1016/j.jstrokecerebrovasdis.2014.12.038. Epub 2015 Mar 25. https://www.ncbi.nlm.nih.gov/pubmed/25817615

30.     da Silva AA, de Mello RG, Schaan CW, Fuchs FD, Redline S, Fuchs SC. Sleep duration and mortality in the elderly: a systematic review with meta-analysis. BMJ Open. 2016 Feb 17;6(2):e008119. doi: 10.1136/bmjopen-2015-008119..

31.     Mims KN, Kirsch D. Sleep and Stroke. Sleep Med Clin. 2016 Mar;11(1):39-51. doi: 10.1016/j.jsmc.2015.10.009. Epub 2016 Jan 9. https://www.ncbi.nlm.nih.gov/pubmed/26972032

32.     https://www.ted.com/talks/russell_foster_why_do_we_sleep Russell Foster. Ted Talk: Why Do We Sleep?

33.     Lao XQ, Liu X, Deng HB, Chan TC, Ho KF, Wang F, Vermeulen R, Tam T, Wong MC, Tse LA, Chang LY, Yeoh EK. Sleep quality, sleep duration, and the risk of coronary heart disease: a prospective cohort study with 60,586 adults. J Clin Sleep Med.2018;14(1):109–11

34     Bin YS. Is sleep quality more important than sleep duration for public health? Sleep. 2016;39(9):1629–1630. [PubMed Central] [PubMed]

35.     Yang TC, Park K. To what extent do sleep quality and duration mediate the effect of perceived discrimination on health? Evidence from Philadelphia. J Urban Health. 2015;92(6):1024–1037. [PubMed Central] PubMed

36.     St-Onge MP, Roberts A, Shechter A, Choudhury AR. Fiber and saturated fat are associated with sleep arousals and slow wave sleep. J Clin Sleep Med 2016;12(1):19–24. http://jcsm.aasm.org/viewabstract.aspx?pid=30412

37.     Karklin A, Driver HS, Buffenstein R, authors. Restricted energy intake affects nocturnal body temperature and sleep patterns. Am J Clin Nutr. 1994;59:346–9. [PubMed]

38.     Crispim CA, Zimberg IZ, dos Reis BG, Diniz RM, Tufik S, de Mello MT, authors. Relationship between food intake and sleep pattern in healthy individuals. J Clin Sleep Med. 2011;7:659–64. [PubMed Central]

39.     Lao XQ, Liu X, Deng HB, Chan TC, Ho KF, Wang F, Vermeulen R, Tam T, Wong MC, Tse LA, Chang LY, Yeoh EK. Sleep quality, sleep duration, and the risk of coronary heart disease: a prospective cohort study with 60,586 adults. J Clin Sleep Med.2018;14(1):109–11

40.     Bin YS. Is sleep quality more important than sleep duration for public health? Sleep. 2016;39(9):1629–1630. [PubMed Central] [PubMed]

41.     Yang TC, Park K. To what extent do sleep quality and duration mediate the effect of perceived discrimination on health? Evidence from Philadelphia. J Urban Health. 2015;92(6):1024–1037. [PubMed Central][PubMed

42.     St-Onge MP, Roberts A, Shechter A, Choudhury AR. Fiber and saturated fat are associated with sleep arousals and slow wave

sleep. J Clin Sleep Med 2016;12(1):19–24. http://jcsm.aasm.org/viewabstract.aspx?pid=30412

43.    Karklin A, Driver HS, Buffenstein R, authors. Restricted energy intake affects nocturnal body temperature and sleep patterns. Am J Clin Nutr. 1994;59:346–9. [PubMed]

44.    Crispim CA, Zimberg IZ, dos Reis BG, Diniz RM, Tufik S, de Mello MT, authors. Relationship between food intake and sleep pattern in healthy individuals. J Clin Sleep Med. 2011;7:659–64. [PubMed Central]

45.    J Altern Complement Med. 2010 Nov;16(11):1145-52. doi: 10.1089/acm.2010.0007. Epub 2010 Aug 19. 3. [PubMed] https://www.ncbi.nlm.nih.gov/pubmed/20722471

46.    Mandolesi, L., Polverino, A., Montuori, S., Foti, F., Ferraioli, G., Sorrentino, P., & Sorrentino, G. (2018). Effects of Physical Exercise on Cognitive Functioning and Wellbeing: Biological and Psychological Benefits. Frontiers in Psychology, 9, 509. http://doi.org/10.3389/fpsyg.2018.00509

47.    https://www.ncbi.nlm.nih.gov/pmc/articles/PMC5934999/ Weinberg R. S., Gould D. (2015). Foundations of sport and exercise psychology, 6th Edn.Champaign, IL: Human Kinetics. [PubMed]

48.    Fernandes J., Arida R. M., Gomez-Pinilla F. (2017). Physical exercise as an epigenetic modulator of brain plasticity and cognition. Neurosci. Biobehav. Rev. 80, 443–456. 10.1016/j.neubiorev.2017.06.012    [PubMed] https://www.ncbi.nlm.nih.gov/pubmed/28666827

49.    Farioli-Vecchioli S., Sacchetti S., di Robilant N. V., Cutuli D. (2018). The role of physical exercise and omega-3 fatty acids in depressive illness in the elderly. Curr. Neuropharmacol. 16, 308–326. [PubMed] https://www.ncbi.nlm.nih.gov/pubmed/28901279

50.    McNulty, J K. "Forgiveness Increases the Likelihood of Subsequent Partner Transgressions in Marriage." Advances in Pediatrics., U.S. National Library of Medicine, Dec. 2010, www.ncbi.nlm.nih.gov/pubmed/21171779.

51.    Russell, V M, et al. "'You're Forgiven, but Don't Do It Again!' Direct Partner Regulation Buffers the Costs of Forgiveness." Advances in Pediatrics., U.S. National Library of Medicine, www.ncbi.nlm.nih.gov/pubmed/29708364.

52.    Takaku, S. "The Effects of Apology and Perspective Taking on Interpersonal Forgiveness: a Dissonance-Attribution Model of Interpersonal Forgiveness." Advances in Pediatrics., U.S. National Library of Medicine, Aug. 2001, www.ncbi.nlm.nih.gov/pubmed/11577848.

53.    J Altern Complement Med. 2010 Nov;16(11):1145-52. doi: 10.1089/acm.2010.0007. Epub 2010 Aug 19. 3. [PubMed] https://www.ncbi.nlm.nih.gov/pubmed/20722471

54.    Mandolesi, L., Polverino, A., Montuori, S., Foti, F., Ferraioli, G., Sorrentino, P., & Sorrentino, G. (2018). Effects of Physical Exercise on Cognitive Functioning and Wellbeing: Biological and Psychological Benefits. Frontiers in Psychology, 9, 509. http://doi.org/10.3389/fpsyg.2018.00509

55.    https://www.ncbi.nlm.nih.gov/pmc/articles/PMC5934999/ Weinberg R. S., Gould D. (2015). Foundations of sport and exercise psychology, 6th Edn.Champaign, IL: Human Kinetics. [PubMed]

56.    Fernandes J., Arida R. M., Gomez-Pinilla F. (2017). Physical exercise as an epigenetic modulator of brain plasticity and cognition. Neurosci. Biobehav. Rev. 80, 443–456. 10.1016/j.neubiorev.2017.06.012    [PubMed] https://www.ncbi.nlm.nih.gov/pubmed/28666827

57.    Farioli-Vecchioli S., Sacchetti S., di Robilant N. V., Cutuli D. (2018). The role of physical exercise and omega-3 fatty acids in depressive illness in the elderly. Curr. Neuropharmacol. 16, 308–326. [PubMed] https://www.ncbi.nlm.nih.gov/pubmed/28901279

58. Health United States Report 2016. https://www.cdc.gov/nchs/data/hus/hus16.pdf

59. "Physical Activity, Aging, and Physiological Function." American Journal of Physiology-Endocrinology and Metabolism, www.physiology.org/doi/abs/10.1152/physiol.00029.2016.

60. Ideno, Y, et al. "Blood Pressure-Lowering Effect of Shinrin-Yoku (Forest Bathing): a Systematic Review and Meta-Analysis." BMC Complementary and Alternative Medicine., U.S. National Library of Medicine, 16 Aug. 2017, www.ncbi.nlm.nih.gov/pubmed/28814305.

61. Booth FW, Roberts CK, Laye MJ. Lack of exercise is a major cause of chronic diseases. Compr Physiol 2: 1143-1211, 2012. https://www.physiology.org/servlet/linkout?suffix=B9&dbid=8&doi=10.1152%2Fphysiol.00029.2016&key=23798298

62. Garcia-Valles, Rebeca, et al. "Life-Long Spontaneous Exercise Does Not Prolong Lifespan but Improves Health Span in Mice." Longevity & Healthspan, BioMed Central, 16 Sept. 2013, longevityandhealthspan.biomedcentral.com/articles/10.1186/2046-2395-2-14.

63. Seals DR, Justice JN, LaRocca TJ.Physiological geroscience: targeting function to increase healthspan and achieve optimal longevity. J Physiol 594: 2001-2024, 2016.

64. Diaz, Keith M., et al. "Patterns of Sedentary Behavior and Mortality in U.S. Middle-Aged and Older Adults: A National Cohort Study." Annals of Internal Medicine, American College of Physicians, 3 Oct. 2017, annals.org/aim/article-abstract/2653704/pat-

terns-sedentary-behavior-mortality-u-s-middle-aged-older-adults.

65. Lautenschlager NT, Cox KL, Flicker L, Foster JK, van Bockxmeer FM, Xiao J, Greenop KR, Almeida OP.Effect of physical activity on cognitive function in older adults at risk for Alzheimer disease: a randomized trial.JAMA 300: 1027-1037, 2008. https://jamanetwork.com/journals/jama/fullarticle/182502

66. Li, Q, et al. "A Day Trip to a Forest Park Increases Human Natural Killer Activity and the Expression of Anti-Cancer Proteins in Male Subjects." Journal of Biological Regulators and Homeostatic Agents., U.S. National Library of Medicine, ncbi.nlm.nih.gov/pubmed/20487629.

67. Ulrich R.S., Addoms D.L. Psychological and recreational benefits of a residential park. Leis. Res. 1981;13:43–65.

68. Li, Q, et al. "A Day Trip to a Forest Park Increases Human Natural Killer Activity and the Expression of Anti-Cancer Proteins in Male Subjects." Journal of Biological Regulators and Homeostatic Agents., U.S. National Library of Medicine, ncbi.nlm.nih.gov/pubmed/20487629.

69. Tsao, Tsung-Ming, et al. "Health Effects of a Forest Environment on Natural Killer Cells in Humans: an Observational Pilot Study." Oncotarget, Impact Journals, 14 Mar. 2018, www.oncotarget.com/index.php?journal=oncotarget&page=article&op=view&path[]=24741.3.

70. Li, Qing. Forest Bathing: How Trees Can Help You Find Health and Happiness. Viking, 2018.

71. Ideno, Y, et al. "Blood Pressure-Lowering Effect of Shinrin-Yoku (Forest Bathing): a Systematic Review and Meta-Analysis." BMC Complementary and Alternative Medicine., U.S. National Library of Medicine, 16 Aug. 2017, ncbi.nlm.nih.gov/pubmed/28814305.

72. Ulrich R.S., Simons R.F., Losito B.D., Fiorito E., Miles M.A., Zelson M. Stress recovery during exposure to natural and urban environments. Environ. Psychol. 1991;11:201–230. doi: 10.1016/S0272-4944(05)80184-7. [Cross Ref]

73. Ulrich R.S. View through a window may influence recovery from surgery. 1984;224:420–421. doi: 10.1126/science.6143402. [PubMed] [Cross Ref]

9. Kaplan R., Kaplan S. The Experience of Nature: A Psychological Perspective.Cambridge University Press; Cambridge, UK: 1989. pp. 177–200.

74. Kaplan S. The restorative benefits of nature: Toward an integrative framework. Environ. Psychol. 1995;15:169–182. doi: 10.1016/0272-4944(95)90001-2. [Cross Ref]

75. Park B.J., Tsunetsugu Y., Kasetani T., Kagawa T., Miyazaki Y. The physiological effects of Shinrin-yoku (taking in the forest atmosphere or forest bathing): Evidence from field experiments in 24 forests across Japan. Health Prev. Med. 2010;15:18–26. doi: 10.1007/s12199-009-0086-9.[PMC free article][PubMed] [Cross Ref]

76. Lee J., Park B.J., Tsunetsugu Y., Ohira T., Kagawa T., Miyazaki Y. Effect of forest bathing on physiological and psychological responses in young Japanese male subjects. Public Health. 2011;125:93–100. doi: 10.1016/j.puhe.2010.09.005. [PubMed][Cross Ref]

77. Lee J., Tsunetsugu Y., Takayama N., Park B.J., Li Q., Song C., Komatsu M., Ikei H., Tyrväinen L., Kagawa T., et al. Influence of forest therapy on cardiovascular relaxation in young adults. Based Complement. Altern. Med. 2014 doi: 10.1155/2014/834360. [PMC free article][PubMed] [Cross Ref]

78. Tsunetsugu Y., Lee J., Park B.J., Tyrväinen L., Kagawa T., Miyazaki Y. Physiological and psychological effects of viewing urban forest landscapes assessed by multiple measurements. Urban Plan. 2013;113:90–93. doi: 10.1016/j.landurbplan.2013.01.014. [Cross Ref]

79. Park B.J., Kasetani T., Morikawa T., Tsunetsugu Y., Kagawa T., Miyazaki Y. Physiological effects of forest recreation in a young conifer forest in Hinokage Town, Japan. Fenn. 2009;43:291–301. doi: 10.14214/sf.213.

80. Rioux, J G, and C Ritenbaugh. "Narrative review of yoga intervention clinical trials including weight-Related outcomes." Alternative therapies in health and medicine., U.S. National Library of Medicine, www.ncbi.nlm.nih.gov/pubmed/23709458.

81. Publishing, Harvard Health. "Yoga for a better sex life?" Harvard Health, www.health.harvard.edu/healthbeat/yoga-for-a-better-sex-life.

82. Lau, C, et al. "Effects of a 12-Week Hatha Yoga Intervention on Cardiorespiratory Endurance, Muscular Strength and Endurance, and Flexibility in Hong Kong Chinese Adults: A Controlled Clinical Trial." Evidence-Based complementary and alternative medicine: eCAM., U.S. National Library of Medicine, www.ncbi.nlm.nih.gov/pubmed/26167196.

83. Manchanda, S C, and K Madan. "Yoga and meditation in cardiovascular disease." Clinical research in cardiology: official journal of the German Cardiac Society., U.S. National Library of Medicine, Sept. 2014, www.ncbi.nlm.nih.gov/pubmed/24464106.

84. Praveena, SM, et al. "Yoga Offers Cardiovascular Protection in Early Postmenopausal Women." International journal of yoga., U.S. National Library of Medicine, www.ncbi.nlm.nih.gov/pubmed/29343929.

85.      Lim, Sung-Ah, and Kwang-Jo Cheong. "Regular Yoga Practice Improves Antioxidant Status, Immune Function, and Stress Hormone Releases in Young Healthy People: A Randomized, Double-Blind, Controlled Pilot Study." The Journal of Alternative and Complementary Medicine, vol. 21, no. 9, 2015, pp. 530–538., doi:10.1089/acm.2014.0044.

86.      Hartfiel N, Havenhand J, Khalsa SB, et al. The effectiveness of yoga for the improvement of well-being and resilience to stress in the workplace. Scand J Work Environ Health 2011;37:70–76.

87.      Michalsen A, Grossman P, Acil A, et al. Rapid stress reduction and anxiolysis among distressed women as a consequence of a three-month intensive yoga program. Med Sci Monitor 2005;11: CR555–561.

88.      Ross A, Friedmann E, Bevans M, Thomas S. National survey of yoga practitioners: mental and physical health benefits. Complement Ther Med 2013;21:313–323.

88.      Nagaraja AS, Armaiz-Pena GN, Lutgendorf SK, Sood AK. Why stress is BAD for cancer patients. J Clin Invest 2013; 123:558–560.

Kovacic T, Zagoricnik M, Kovacic M. Impact of relaxation training according to the Yoga In Daily Life(R) system on anxiety after breast cancer surgery. J Complement Integr Med 2013;10.

89.      Mustian KM, Sprod LK, Janelsins M, et al. Multicenter, randomized controlled trial of yoga for sleep quality among cancer survivors. J Clin Oncology 2013;31:3233–3241

## BOOKS TO INSPIRE

Adele, Deborah. The Yamas & Niyamas: Exploring Yogas Ethical Practice. On-Word Bound Books, 2009.

Alcantara, Margarita, and Tom Bingham. Chakra Healing: a Beginners Guide to Self-Healing Techniques That Balance the Chakras. Fall River Press, 2019.

Alexander, Eben. Proof of Heaven: a Neurosurgeons Journey into the Afterlife. Large Print Press, 2013.

Barrett, Jayme, and Weihua Xue. Liao Zhai Zhi Y.  Fengshui Your Life. Zhongguo. She Hui Chu Ban She, 2004.

Burchard, Brendon. High Performance Habits: How Extraordinary People Become That Way. Hay House, Inc., 2017.

Carrera, Jaganath. Inside the Yoga Sutras: a Comprehensive Sourcebook for the Study and Practice of Patanjalis Yoga Sutras. Integral Yoga Publications, 2006.

Chapman, Gary D. The 5 Love Languages. Northfield Pub., 2015.

Chopra, Deepak. Ageless Body, Timeless Mind. Rider, 1998.

Chopra, Deepak. Seven Spiritual Laws of Success. Amber-Allen, 2007.

Chopra, Deepak. Reinventing the Body, Resurrecting the Soul: How to Create a New Self. Rider, 2010.

Chopra, Deepak. Reinventing the Body, Resurrecting the Soul: How to Create a New You. Three Rivers Press, 2010.

Clear, James. Atomic Habits: an Easy & Proven Way to Build Good Habits & Break Bad Ones. Avery, an Imprint of Penguin Random House, 2018.

Frankl, V. E. Man's Search for Meaning. Pocket, 1946.

Greger, Michael. How Not to Die. Pan Books, 2017.

Kalanithi, Paul, and Abraham Verghese. When Breath Becomes Air. Vintage, 2018.

Kondō Marie, and Cathy Hirano. The Life-Changing Magic of Tidying up: the Japanese Art of Decluttering and Organizing. Thorndike Press, a Part of Gale, Cengage Learning, 2015.

Loomis, Carol. Tap Dancing to Work: Warren Buffett on Practically Everything, 1966-2013: a Fortune Magazine Book. Portfolio Penguin, 2014

Mihm, Dorothea, and Annette Bopp. Die Sieben Geheimnisse Guten Sterbens: Erfahrungen einer Buddhistischen Palliativschwester. Goldmann, 2017.

Robbins, Anthony. Awaken the Giant Within: How to Take Immediate Control of Your Mental, Emotional, Physical & Financial Destiny! Simon & Schuster Paperbacks, 2013.

Rock, David. Your Brain at Work. 2009.

Singer, Michael A. The Untethered Soul: the Journey beyond Yourself. New Harbinger Publications, Inc., 2013.

Tolle, Eckhart. Stillness Speaks. Hodder, 2006.

Tolle, Eckhart. A New Earth: Awakening to Your Lifes Purpose. Penguin Books, 2016.

Tolle, Eckhart. The Power of Now: a Guide to Spiritual Enlightenment. Hachette Australia, 2018.

Voss, Christopher, and Tahl Raz. Never Split the Difference: Negotiating as If Your Life Depended on It. RH Business Books, 2016.

Zukav, Gary, et al. The Seat of the Soul. Simon and Schuster, 1989.

Voss, Christopher, and Tahl Raz. Never Split the Difference: Negotiating as If Your Life Depended on It. RH

www.ingramcontent.com/pod-product-compliance
Lightning Source LLC
Chambersburg PA
CBHW060759270326
41926CB00002B/34